The IBD Nutrition Book

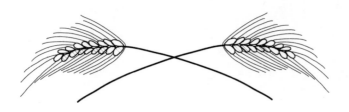

The IBD Nutrition Book

Jan K. Greenwood, R.D.N., C.N.S.D.

John Wiley & Sons, Inc.
New York • Chichester • Brisbane • Toronto • Singapore

In recognition of the importance of preserving what has been written, it is a policy of John Wiley & Sons, Inc., to have books of enduring value published in the United States printed on acid-free paper, and we exert our best efforts to that end.

Library of Congress Cataloging-in-Publication Data

Greenwood, Jan K., 1956–
    The IBD nutrition book / by Jan K. Greenwood.
      p. cm.
    Includes index.
    ISBN 0-471-54630-5 (pbk. : alk. paper)
    1. Inflammatory bowel diseases–Diet therapy.   2. Inflammatory
bowel diseases–Nutritional aspects. I. Title.
    RC862.I53G74   1992
    616.3'440654–dc20   91-41117

Printed in the United States of America
10 9 8 7 6 5 4 3 2 1

Printed and bound by Courier Companies, Inc.

*Dedicated to the many individuals
with inflammatory bowel disease
who provided me with the inspiration for this book.*

ACKNOWLEDGMENTS

In deep appreciation of my husband, Glen, whose constant encouragement and support made this work an enjoyable experience.

Thank you to my colleagues at Vancouver General Hospital who, through example, encourage excellence in nutrition and patient care.

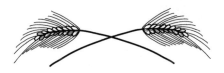

Contents

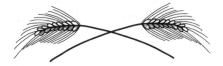

Introduction

The term *inflammatory bowel disease* (IBD) refers to two chronic inflammatory conditions: Crohn's disease and ulcerative colitis. Although two distinct diseases, Crohn's disease and ulcerative colitis are similar in that they are characterized by a chronic (recurring or occurring over a long period of time) inflammation involving various areas and layers of the gastrointestinal tract. The gastrointestinal tract is the organ of nutrient digestion and absorption. It is the disruption of this organ by inflammation and the associated symptoms of pain, nausea, and diarrhea that contribute to the high incidence of poor nutrition associated with these diseases. For various reasons, much confusion exists as to what can and should be eaten by the individual with IBD. Since preventing and correcting poor nutrition is a key component in the overall care of the individual with Crohn's disease or ulcerative colitis, it is essential that good nutrition and the structure of a proper diet be clearly understood by all individuals with these diseases.

This book was written to guide the adult with IBD along the often confusing road of diet and nutrition. The topics of normal digestion and absorption, key essential nutrients and their role in relationship to IBD, special diets, and much more have been addressed in the following pages. Special sections that specifically address the nutrition concerns of preschoolers to adolescents and women of child-bearing years have also been included. The Glossary is to be used as a quick resource to clarify the nutritional and medical terms. A special recipe section has been included to stimulate the appetite and to provide further guidance. To accommodate both American and Canadian readers, measurements have been stated in both metric and imperial units. Any differences between the American and Canadian nutrition recommendations have been noted.

The information in this book is intended to reinforce the importance of eating well, to provide the practical knowledge necessary to make wise food choices, and to promote the achievement of good nutrition. Readers are encouraged to seek additional nutrition advice from a registered dietitian if they require more information and direction. The section on resources provides instruction on how to contact a registered dietitian directly.

The IBD Nutrition Book

I

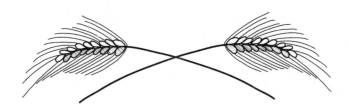

Nutrition and Inflammatory Bowel Disease

1

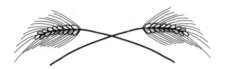

The Basics of Nutrition

NUTRITION

The definition of nutrition can be basically stated as the relationship of food to the well-being of the body. Good nutrition is the state that exists when the body has been receiving the proper amounts of the nutrients that it needs to function properly. In short, good nutrition is essential to good health. In a well-nourished state, the body functions efficiently in carrying out essential body processes, providing for growth and reproduction, resisting infection, and repairing body damage. Malnutrition—the state of being poorly nourished—develops when the body does not receive the needed amounts of the various essential nutrients for a significant length of time. In a malnourished state, the body does not work efficiently, general energy level and work efficiency declines, the ability to resist infection and to heal is reduced, and the process of growth and development becomes impaired. If the state of malnutrition is not corrected, the body may deteriorate to a point where the general state of health is seriously affected and the ability to respond to medical therapy is greatly impeded.

In IBD, malnutrition is a well-documented common consequence of the disease process. Crohn's disease tends to carry a higher risk of malnutrition than ulcerative colitis, but with both diseases, poor nutrition is prevalent. A number of nutritional deficiencies have been reported in a significant percentage of hospitalized individuals with IBD. These include protein-energy malnutrition (an insufficiency of both protein and energy leading to weight loss and poor healing); various vitamin deficiencies, including vitamin A, vitamin D, vitamin C, folic acid, and B_{12}; metabolic bone diseases such as osteoporosis (a condition in which a reduction in the amount of bone occurs) and osteomalacia (a condition in which the bone becomes softer); and mineral deficiencies such as iron and zinc. These same deficiencies are thought to exist to a lesser extent in individuals with IBD outside of the hospital setting.

Although there is often no single identifiable cause of malnutrition in IBD, the most common contributing factor is simply an inadequate dietary intake. This can result from an inability to eat or a loss of appetite when symptoms of pain, nausea, and diarrhea are present. Also, diet can be poor because of a fear of eating, thereby precipitating the disease or its symptoms. Overly restrictive diets without supplementation, either followed by necessity or self-prescribed, can also contribute to an overall inadequate nutritional intake. Other contributory factors include the following:

1. Malabsorption

   - Reduced absorptive surface from disease or surgical resection (surgical removal)
   - Bacterial overgrowth in the gastrointestinal tract, which interferes with nutrient utilization

2. Increased secretion and nutrient loss

   - Protein-losing enteropathy (loss of protein through the inflamed bowel wall)
   - Loss of electrolytes and minerals because of diarrhea
   - Loss of blood from the bowel

3. Drug(s) affecting nutrients

   - Prednisone—reduces calcium absorption and increases protein breakdown
   - Sulfasalazine—reduces folate absorption
   - Cholestyramine—interferes with fat-soluble vitamin absorption

4. Increased utilization and increased requirements

- Fever and infection—increase nutrient needs
- Energy requirements—increase to promote weight gain

There is no documentation to support the theory that following a diet which includes or avoids certain foods affects the disease process. No food can initiate active disease or induce a remission (the period of inactive disease). However, attaining and maintaining a good nutritional state is essential. Being well-nourished greatly improves the ability to fight infection, heal, and respond to medical therapy. Unfortunately, this is easier said than done, especially in active disease, when pain, nausea, anorexia (loss of appetite for food), and diarrhea may be present to interfere with nutrition. Knowledge, motivation, and an emphasis on wise food choices at all times will help ensure a well-nourished body that is well armed to meet any nutritional challenge.

DIGESTION AND ABSORPTION

Digestion is a series of physical and chemical events by which food is taken into the body and is broken down in preparation for absorption from the intestinal tract into the blood stream. The digestive system extends from the mouth to the anus and is highly organized and regulated. Each section of the digestive system has a specific role to play in nutrient absorption. (Refer to Figure 1.) The *mouth* receives the food and reduces it in size and structure by the action of chewing and by mixing with saliva, which contains digestive enzymes (proteins that facilitate chemical reactions). The *esophagus*, a hollow muscular tube, transports food from the mouth to the *stomach*, an expandable sack that receives the food. Through churning action and the addition of enzymes and strong acid, the food is further broken down into a liquid. At regular intervals, a small amount of this liquid mass is released into the *small intestine*. The small intestine consists of the duodenum, the jejunum, and the ileum. The *pancreas* produces secretions required for the digestion and absorption of food. The secretions of the pancreas are released into the duodenum in response to the presence of food there. The *liver* has many functions, but its main process in digestion is the production and excretion of bile salts. Bile salts aid in the digestion of fats by acting as a detergent. The *gallbladder* stores and concentrates bile salts when they are not immediately required for the digestion of food. The duodenum, the jejunum, and the ileum absorb all the nutrients of digestion through specialized fingerlike projections called villi. Nutrient absorption is well regulated to accommodate the many kinds of nutrients and the various amounts needed by the body. Once absorbed as nutrients, they pass into the blood for delivery to the cells of the body. The undigested material moves from the small

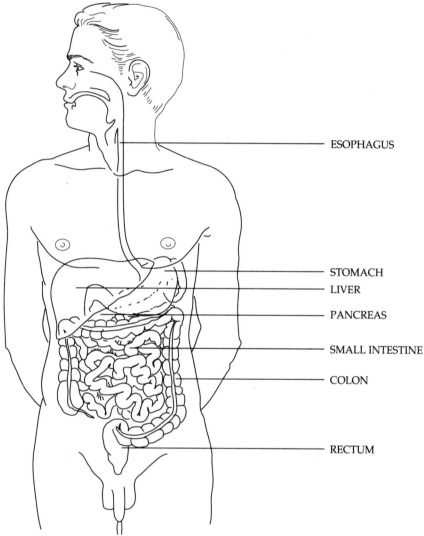

ESOPHAGUS

STOMACH

LIVER

PANCREAS

SMALL INTESTINE

COLON

RECTUM

Figure 1   The gastrointestinal tract.

intestine into the *colon*, also referred to as the large intestine, where water and electrolytes such as sodium and potassium are absorbed. At the end of the large intestine, the *rectum* functions as a temporary storage site for feces (the waste matter excreted from the bowel, consisting of unabsorbed food, water, bacteria, and intestinal secretions) before it is passed from the body.

From this description, it is clear that the small intestine is the key area of nutrient digestion and absorption. If disease or surgical resection affects a significant portion of this area, the risk of nutrient malabsorption (poor or disordered absorption) and malnutrition is increased. On the other hand, disease or surgical resection of all or part of the large intestine is not usually associated with significant malabsorption unless combined with disease or resection of the small intestine. Because it is Crohn's disease, and not ulcerative colitis, that may affect the small intestine, Crohn's disease is more often associated with malabsorption and malnutrition. This is not to imply that malnutrition does not occur in ulcerative colitis or that nutrition is not as important. For both diseases, a poor diet, especially during active disease, can lead to significant malnutrition. Hence, good nutrition practices followed on a daily basis are an essential component of care for both Crohn's disease and ulcerative colitis.

ESSENTIAL NUTRIENTS AND THEIR FUNCTION

Nutrients are the chemical components of food that the body requires to perform the various activities associated with living. There are more than 45 essential nutrients, and they are grouped into the categories listed below. Those nutrients required daily in relatively large quantities, such as grams, are called *macronutrients*. These include protein, fat, and carbohydrate. Nutrients required in smaller amounts, such as milligrams or micrograms, are called *micronutrients*. These include vitamins and minerals. Regardless of the amount required by the body, each nutrient has a specific role to play in good health. Energy (the fuel required by the body to power body processes) is derived from protein, fat, and carbohydrate. Vitamins and minerals do not provide energy but aid in the chemical reactions that allow the conversion of protein, fat, and carbohydrate to energy. All nutrients are dependent on the others; none function totally independently. The following is a partial list of the essential nutrients and their functions.

MACRONUTRIENTS

Protein	Builds and repairs all body tissues
	Builds antibodies (blood components that fight infection)
	Builds enzymes and some hormones
Fat	A concentrated energy source
	Supplies essential fatty acids
	Aids in the absorption of fat-soluble vitamins
Carbohydrate	The body's main source of energy
	Spares protein

Water   Necessary for adequate fluid balance
                         Involved in body temperature regulation ,

MICRONUTRIENTS

Vitamins

Thiamin   Assists energy release from carbohydrate
                         Aids in normal growth and appetite

Riboflavin   Maintains healthy skin and normal vision
                         Maintains normal function of the nervous system
                         Releases energy to body cells during metabolism (the
                            sum total of all chemical reactions that take place in
                            living cells)

Niacin   Aids normal growth and development
                         Maintains a normal nervous system and digestive tract

Pyridoxine   Aids in the utilization of protein

Folacin   Aids in red blood cell formation
(Folic Acid)

Vitamin B_{12} Aids in red blood cell formation
(Cobalamin)   Maintains healthy functioning of the nervous system and
                            gastrointestinal tract

Biotin   Functions in the metabolism of fats and carbohydrates

Pantothenic acid   Involved in the utilization of macronutrients in energy
                            production

Vitamin C   Maintains healthy gums and teeth
                         Maintains strong blood vessel walls

Vitamin A   Aids in normal bone and tooth formation
                         Aids in normal vision
                         Maintains the health of skin and membranes

Vitamin D   Aids in the absorption and utilization of calcium in the
                            formation and maintenance of strong bones and teeth

Vitamin E   Maintains health of membranes

Vitamin K   Required for normal blood clotting

Minerals

Sodium	Involved in body fluid distribution and nerve function
Potassium	Involved in body fluid distribution Required for proper nerve transmission and muscle contraction Plays a role in protein and carbohydrate metabolism
Chloride	Helps maintain the body's acid-base balance
Calcium	Aids in the formation and maintenance of strong bones and teeth Aids healthy nerve function and normal blood clotting
Iron	An important component of hemoglobin (the red blood cell constituent that transports oxygen and carbon dioxide)
Phosphorus	Aids in the formation and maintenance of strong bones and teeth Regulates the release of energy
Magnesium	Aids in the formation and maintenance of strong bones and teeth Aids in normal muscle and nerve function
Zinc	Required for normal growth and development
Iodine	Aids in the function of the thyroid gland
Copper	Involved in hemoglobin and connective tissue formation
Fluoride	Important for strong teeth
Chromium	Aids the action of insulin (the hormone that helps cells take up sugar from the blood and use it for energy)
Selenium	Helps protect vitamin E
Manganese	Plays a role in brain function
Molybdenum, lithium, cobalt, boron, nickel, vanadium, silicon	Possibly necessary in very small quantities; the role of some of these elements remains unclear

MEETING NUTRIENT NEEDS USING FOOD GUIDES

In order to maintain the body in a healthy state, all essential nutrients must be provided in the proper amounts and on a regular basis. In the United States, the nutrition recommendations are called the Recommended Dietary Allowances (RDAs), whereas in Canada, the nutrition recommendations are called the Recommended Nutrient Intakes (RNIs). Both of these recommendations outline the quantity of each nutrient thought to be sufficient to meet most healthy individuals' needs based on age, sex, body size, activity, and diet. The RDA and the RNI should not be viewed as a specific nutrient requirement that must be taken daily to avoid a deficiency, but an amount that allows for individual differences and therefore a generous statement of general need. Although expressed on a daily basis, both the RDA and the RNI should be regarded as the average recommended daily intake over a period of time, such as a week. Although the RDA and the RNI often exceed the requirement to maintain health in already healthy individuals, in IBD or in any disease state where nutrient losses or needs are increased, the RDA and RNI may be inadequate. The RDA and the RNI are very similar but small differences do exist.

The RDA and the RNI, because of degree of detail, are not used in everyday practice to plan meals or to evaluate the adequacy of one's diet. There are several food guides available that provide a more practical means to plan well-balanced diets and hence meet nutrient needs. In the United States, the food guide is called the *Four Food Groups*, or simply the Basic Four. In Canada, the food guide is referred to as *Canada's Food Guide*. Both of these guidelines help take the detail

Examples of Recommended Dietary Allowances (RDAs) and Recommended Nutrient Intakes (RNIs)

Age (years)	Sex	Weight (kg/lb)	Protein (g/day)	Vitamin C (mg/day)	Folacin (μ/day)	Calcium (mg/day)	Iron (mg/day)
				RDAs (1989)			
19–24	M	72/160	58	60	200	1200	10
	F	58/128	46	60	180	1200	15
25–50	M	79/174	63	60	200	800	10
	F	63/138	50	60	180	800	15
				RNIs (1990)			
19–24	M	71/156	61	40	220	800	9
	F	58/128	50	30	180	700	13
25–49	M	74/163	64	40	230	800	9
	F	59/130	51	30	185	700	13

and guesswork out of balancing a diet and meeting nutrient needs because it is easier and more practical to think in terms of actual foods than it is to count quantities of nutrients. These guides bring together foods into four groups, according to each food's nutrient composition. Although the exact name and some serving sizes may vary slightly, both guides are very similar. In general, the four food groups are the milk and milk products group; the meat and alternates group; the breads and cereals group; and the fruits and vegetables group. Together the four food groups provide all the nutrients necessary for good health. Each food group has its own unique composition of key nutrients, and, for this reason, the groups are not interchangeable. For example, red meat provides iron but not calcium, whereas milk provides calcium but not iron. Foods contain not just one but a number of nutrients that are often interrelated. For example, one nutrient may aid in the absportion of another. The practice of replacing a food with a vitamin or mineral supplement is not encouraged. As much as possible, nutrients should be obtained from food. When one consumes daily the recommended number of servings of each food group found therein, the Basic Four and Canada's Food Guide will meet most individuals' nutrient needs.

As with the RDA and the RNI, the food guides are based on healthy individuals without disease or altered nutrient requirements. Increased needs must be considered for people with IBD, but these needs can often be met by increasing the serving size or number of servings from each food group. As previously stated, nutrient needs should be met through a well-balanced diet. However, in some situations, nutrient requirements may necessitate the use of a supplement. Individuals should not take any vitamin or mineral supplement without consulting their physician and registered dietitian, since taking too much of any nutrient can be hazardous. Refer to the section on vitamin and mineral supplements for further discussion.

The basic four contains a fifth group that includes fats, sweets, and alcohol. Canada's Food Guide does not have a specific group for these foods, but they are generally acknowledged as "extras." These foods are sources of energy but are not key sources of nutrients. Foods should be chosen from this last group only when nutrient needs have been met as outlined in the food guide. This does not mean that these foods should never be eaten. For example, fats are an excellent source of energy, and for individuals who are underweight, they are an easy way to aid in weight gain. Sweets are a tasty and ready source of energy and, when incorporated into the diet, often improve total energy intake, especially when appetite is poor. The use of a well-balanced diet based on the food guides with fats and sweets added as an energy source is encouraged.

The food guides do not address meal frequency. Some individuals prefer to consume three meals per day whereas others consume smaller meals more frequently. The most important requirement is that meals be eaten regularly throughout the day, rather than relying on one large meal in the evening. The practice of consuming one large evening meal may lead to a limited and unbalanced diet, weakness during the day, and abdominal bloating and cramping following the meal. If you are following such a dietary regimen in order to control daytime bowel movements, talk to your physician. Various medications are available that can help reduce stool frequency (fecal discharge from the bowel) and allow you to eat regularly during the day.

The RDA and RNI and food guide groups are frequently referenced throughout this book. You are encouraged to consult the food guide food groups for guidance in maintaining a well-balanced diet. In this book, the names of the food groups and serving sizes have been altered slightly from the individual food guides in an attempt to accommodate both American and Canadian readers. You are encouraged to obtain a copy of the food guide used in your country and to utilize it in establishing your well-balanced diet. Your physician or registered dietitian can assist you in obtaining a copy of the food guide.

THE FOOD GROUPS—KEY NUTRIENTS

Each food group supplies a unique combination of key nutrients. When foods are chosen in the recommended number of servings from each group, all daily nutrient needs can be met. The following table outlines the key nutrients provided by each food group.

Milk Group	+	Meat/ Alternate Group	+	Bread/Cereal Group	+	Fruit/Vegetable Group	=	Balanced Diet
Protein		Protein		Protein				Protein
Fat		Fat						Fat
				Carbohydrate		Carbohydrate		Carbohydrate
		Thiamin		Thiamin		Thiamin		Thiamin
Riboflavin		Riboflavin		Riboflavin				Riboflavin
Niacin		Niacin		Niacin				Niacin
Folacin				Folacin		Folacin		Folacin
Vitamin B_{12}		Vitamin B_{12}						Vitamin B_{12}
						Vitamin C		Vitamin C
Vitamin A		Vitamin A				Vitamin A		Vitamin A
Vitamin D								Vitamin D
Calcium								Calcium
		Iron		Iron		Iron		Iron
		Fiber		Fiber		Fiber		Fiber

FOOD GUIDES—CANADA'S FOOD GUIDE AND THE BASIC FOUR

In Canada, the dietary guide used by individuals to help balance their diet is called *Canada's Food Guide*. In the United States, the dietary guide is referred to as the Basic Four. Both food guides outline four food groups, a recommended number of servings from each group, and the serving sizes required on a daily basis in order to meet nutrient needs. Both guides emphasize variety and the inclusion of a food from each food group at each meal. The following is the guideline for adults.

MILK AND MILK PRODUCTS

Choose 2 servings per day

Examples of one serving:

250 mL (1 cup) whole, skim, 2% milk

175–250 mL ($\frac{3}{4}$–1 cup) yogurt

45 g ($1\frac{1}{2}$ oz) cheddar or process cheese

MEAT AND ALTERNATES

Choose 2 servings per day

Examples of one serving:

60–90 g (2–3 oz) cooked lean meat, poultry, liver or fish

60 mL (4 tbsp) peanut butter

250 mL (1 cup) cooked dried peas or beans

125 mL ($\frac{1}{2}$ cup) nuts or seeds

60 g (2 oz) cheese

2 eggs

FRUITS AND VEGETABLES

Choose 4–5 servings per day (include at least two vegetables)

Examples of one serving:

125 mL ($\frac{1}{2}$ cup) vegetables or fruits

125 mL ($\frac{1}{2}$ cup) juice

1 medium potato, carrot, tomato, peach, apple, orange, or banana

BREADS AND CEREALS

Choose 3–5 servings per day (select enriched and whole grain products)

Examples of one serving:

1 slice of bread

125 mL ($\frac{1}{2}$ cup) cooked cereal

1 roll or muffin

125–175 mL ($\frac{1}{2}$–$\frac{3}{4}$ cup) cooked rice or macaroni

Sample Balanced Diet Using Food Guides

Food Item	Food Group Source
Breakfast	
125 mL ($\frac{1}{2}$ cup) orange juice	1 serving from the fruit/vegetable group
250 mL (1 cup) 2% milk	1 serving from the milk group
2 slices whole-wheat bread	2 servings from the bread/cereal group
10 mL (2 tsp) butter	Extra group*
1 poached egg	$\frac{1}{2}$ serving from the meat/alternate group
Lunch	
250 mL (1 cup) tossed salad	1 serving from the fruit/vegetable group
15 mL (1 tbsp) salad dressing	Extra group*
Cheese sandwich:	
30 g (1 oz) cheese	$\frac{1}{2}$ serving from the meat/alternate group
2 slices whole-wheat bread	2 servings from the bread/cereal group
5–10 mL (1–2 tsp) butter	Extra group*
1 apple	1 serving from the fruit/vegetable group
Snack	
1 multi-grain dinner roll	1 serving from the bread/cereal group
5–10 mL (1–2 tsp) butter	Extra group*
Evening Meal	
250 mL (1 cup) 2% milk	1 serving from the milk group
90 g (3 oz) roast beef	1 serving from the meat/alternate group
1 baked potato	1 serving from the fruit/vegetable group
5–10 mL (1–2 tsp) butter	Extra group*
125 mL ($\frac{1}{2}$ cup) cooked carrots	1 serving from the fruit/vegetable group
125 mL ($\frac{1}{2}$ cup) sherbet	Extra group*

*Extra group = fats, sweets, and alcohol.

ARE YOU MEETING YOUR NUTRIENT NEEDS?

In the columns below, write down all food items you ate yesterday. Divide what was eaten into the four food groups. Check the food guides for groups and serving sizes. Total the number of servings in each column and compare to the recommended number of servings.

Food Eaten	Amount	Milk	Meat	Fruit/Vegetable	Bread/Cereal
Your Servings from Each Group					
Recommended Servings		2	2	4–5	3–5

Did you meet your nutrient needs yesterday? Compare to see which food groups you need to improve.

2

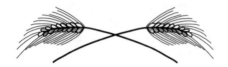

Key Nutrients in Detail

MACRONUTRIENTS

Protein, fat, and carbohydrate are referred to as *macronutrients* because they are required in relatively large amounts in comparison to other nutrients. This does not imply that these nutrients are more important than those nutrients required in smaller amounts; it is simply a means of describing the body's requirements. Unlike vitamins and minerals, macronutrients can be broken down in the body to provide energy. Energy is required to drive many body processes—tissue formation, physical movement, temperature regulation, and much more. In nutrition, food energy is measured in units. In the United States, the unit of measure is the kilocalorie (kcal), often simply referred to as a calorie. In Canada, the unit of measure is the kilojoule (kJ). Macronutrients have many other functions besides supplying energy. The following discussion will review each macronutrient in detail, with an emphasis on their role and relationship with IBD.

Protein

The term *protein* is derived from a Greek word meaning "to take first place." Although all nutrients are important, protein has always been given a special place, since it is a part of every living cell. The functions of protein are numerous. It is used to repair worn-out body tissue resulting from daily "wear and tear," and to build new tissue during periods of growth, such as pregnancy, childhood, and healing. Normal body fluid balance is maintained partially by the various proteins in the blood. These same proteins are important in transporting vitamins and minerals throughout the body. In addition, proteins, in the form of antibodies, play a key role in enabling the body to resist infection.

The requirement for protein varies depending on age, sex, weight, and state of health. Unlike other nutrients, an excess dietary intake is not stored, and protein must thus be consumed on a daily basis. The daily requirement for healthy adults is approximately 0.5 to 1 gram (g) of protein per kilogram (kg) of body weight. As such, the average daily protein requirement for adult males and females of average body weight between the ages of 19 and 24 is approximately 60 g and 45 g, respectively. In individuals with active IBD, the requirement for protein increases. The extra protein is required to repair damaged tissue, replace the protein lost as a result of protein-losing enteropathy, and replace the protein that the body uses as an extra energy source during the active phase of illness. Therefore, during periods when IBD is active, it is reasonable to aim for a daily protein intake of at least 50 percent greater than the RDA or the RNI for healthy adults. This would represent a daily intake of approximately 85 g for males and 70 g for females of average weight. To ensure that the protein is used for important body functions, it is essential that adequate energy be consumed along with it. If inadequate energy is consumed, protein will be used as an energy source and will not be available to repair damaged tissue. For this reason, weight loss during active disease is to be discouraged.

Protein deficiency is quite common in active IBD. Increased losses from the bowel, poor dietary intake, reduced protein synthesis (the process involving the formation of a complex substance from a simpler substance) by the body, and increased needs are all contributing factors. In addition, steroid medications such as prednisone, which are often used to reduce inflammation in active disease, increase the breakdown of body protein. Poor protein status contributes to delayed healing, a decreased resistance to infection, muscle loss, and the development of edema (the collection of unusually large amounts of body fluid in a part of or all of the body and which results in swelling). A good protein intake, especially during and after active disease, is therefore encouraged. Refer to the section on high-protein diet for further information and guidance.

Through the process of digestion, protein in the diet is broken down into more basic units called *amino acids* and absorbed in the upper small intestine. Of the twenty naturally occurring amino acids, nine cannot be made by the human body and must be supplied by the diet. These nine are referred to as essential amino acids. Proteins that contain the correct combination of essential amino acids are referred to as complete protein. Complete protein is found in foods of animal origin such as eggs, milk, cheese, fish, chicken, pork, and beef. An incomplete protein is low or deficient in one or more of the essential amino acids and is found in foods of vegetable origin such as fruit, vegetables, grains, seeds, and legumes such as lentils and peas. This is not meant to imply that vegetable protein is of no value. By combining two or more proteins that together supply all the amino acids, a complete protein can be made available to the body. There are two ways to form complete proteins. First, one can combine an animal protein with a plant protein. An example of this option would be food choices from the milk group combined with foods from the bread/cereal group, as in a meal of milk and cereal. A second method is to combine two or more plant proteins that complement each other and together supply all the essential amino acids. For example, one might combine a food from the meat/alternate group with a food from the bread/cereal group,

Food Sources of Protein

Food Group	Food Item	Serving Size	Protein (g)
Milk group	Milk	250 mL (1 cup)	8
	Yogurt	175–250 mL ($\frac{3}{4}$–1 cup)	8
	Cheese	45 g ($1\frac{1}{2}$ oz)	9–13
Meat/alternate group	Lean meat, fish, poultry (cooked)	60–90 g (2–3 oz)	14–21
	Cottage cheese	125 mL ($\frac{1}{2}$ cup)	15
	Egg	2	12
	Peanut butter	60 mL (4 tbsp)	16
	Nuts, seeds	125 mL ($\frac{1}{2}$ cup)	11–21
	Dried peas, beans, lentils (cooked)	250 mL (1 cup)	12–17
	Tofu	90 g (3 oz)	7
Bread/cereal group	Bread	1 slice	2
	Cooked cereal	125 mL ($\frac{1}{2}$ cup)	2
	Cold cereal	175 mL ($\frac{3}{4}$ cup)	2
	Rice, macaroni (cooked)	125–175 mL ($\frac{1}{2}$–$\frac{3}{4}$ cup)	2
Fruit/vegetable group	Fruit, vegetable, or juice	125 mL ($\frac{1}{2}$ cup)	0.5–1

as in a meal of baked beans and whole-wheat bread. A good rule of thumb is to consume an animal-origin protein at each meal to enhance the protein quality of the meal.

The table on page 19 lists the protein content of selected foods within the food groups of the food guides. The foods listed above the dotted line are sources of complete protein, and those below the line are sources of incomplete protein.

Protein quality is not affected by cooking methods or meal preparation. It is most important that protein-rich foods be handled and stored properly. Proper storage will prevent bacterial contamination and spoilage, which could lead to nutrient destruction or food poisoning or both. Although commercial protein supplements are available, they are most often unnecessary, since protein needs usually can be met by simple dietary manipulation. Supplements should not be used without the advice of your physician and registered dietitian because an excessive intake may affect the requirements of other nutrients. Also, any excess intake of protein above actual needs will simply be used as energy, as the body does not store protein. If you must obtain a higher protein intake, refer to the section on high-protein diets for further information. If you are following a vegetarian diet, especially if you are omitting most or all animal flesh and its products from your diet, you are encouraged to seek further advice from your physician and registered dietitian.

Fat

Although it is not a key source of nutrients, fat serves as a concentrated source of energy. Each gram of fat provides 38 kilojoules (kJ), or 9 kilocalories (kcal), which is more than twice the energy value of an equal amount of protein or carbohydrate. For this reason, fats are of great value when weight gain is desired, especially if appetite is poor. Dietary fat aids in the absorption of the fat soluble vitamins A, D, E, and K; it serves as a source of the essential fatty acid linoleic acid, which is necessary for growth, reproduction, and healthy skin; and it enhances the taste of many foods. To meet these needs, a daily fat intake of 30 to 35 percent of total energy intake is suggested. This means that in an 8400 kJ (2000 kcal) daily diet, there should be 60 to 70 g of fat. If weight gain is not desired, if fat malabsorption is present, or if fat intake is contraindicated for other health reasons such as heart disease, the amount of fat in the diet should be lowered. If weight gain is desired or if there is difficulty in maintaining present weight, the fat intake may need to be increased.

When fat is consumed in the diet, bile is released from the gallbladder. The bile acts on large fat molecules to break them into small particles that can be readily absorbed. Because bile acids are reabsorbed by the body in the terminal ileum (the end section of the ileum), surgical resection or active disease of all or part of the ileum often results in bile acid malabsorption. If bile acid malabsorption is severe, a bile acid deficiency may develop, which reduces the body's ability to absorb fats. If fat is not well digested and absorbed, steatorrhea (an excessive amount of fat in the stool) results. With steatorrhea, the stool will have a high fat content, which causes it to have a foul smell and to float. Nutritionally, fat malabsorption contributes to a loss of energy, fat-soluble vitamins, calcium, and magnesium. If uncorrected, fat malabsorption may cause weight loss and symptoms of vitamin deficiency. If fat malabsorption has been detected, some degree of dietary fat restriction may be necessary. Except in the case of steatorrhea, a restricted-fat diet is not generally required or encouraged for individuals with IBD, since this may impair total energy intake. Refer to the dietary modifications section for further information on restricted fat diets. Inadequate energy intake resulting from the need to restrict dietary fat may be alleviated partially by the use of a commercial dietary supplement. Refer to the section on commercial supplements for a discussion of these products.

The principle sources of fat in the diet can be divided into two groups: visible fat and invisible fat. Visible fat is fat that you can readily see and includes butter, margarine, lard, vegetable oil, the visible fat of meat, and the skin on chicken. Invisible fat is not so readily apparent and is found in such foods as cream, whole milk and its products, cheese, egg yolk, avocado, nuts, and seeds. Food preparation and cooking has no appreciable effect on the nutritional value of fats. However, when fats and oils are exposed to warm, moist air for a period of time, chemical changes occur that produce unpalatable flavors and odors; this unpleasant change is called rancidity. This process can destroy any vitamin A and E present in the food. Therefore, fat-containing foods should be stored in a refrigerator.

If you are required to follow a restricted-fat diet, you are encouraged to seek further advice from your physician and registered dietitian to ensure that you are meeting your nutrient and energy needs.

Carbohydrate

All body processes require energy to function, and carbohydrates serve as a readily available, easily digestible energy source to meet those demands. There are three groups of carbohydrate, based on the number of sugar units making up the carbohydrate—monosaccharides, disaccharides, and polysaccharides. Monosaccharides are single units of sugar, which are readily digested and absorbed. Glucose, required by the body for all metabolic processes, is an example of a monosaccharide. Disaccharides are two sugar units linked together. When broken down by enzymes in the small intestine, two readily absorbable sugars are produced. For example, lactose, or milk sugar, is broken down to yield glucose and galactose. Both monosaccharides and disaccharides are referred to as simple carbohydrates or simple sugars. Polysaccharides, the third group of carbohydrates, are composed of multiple units of sugar; polysaccharides are often referred to as complex carbohydrates. Like disaccharides, polysaccharides must be broken down in the gastrointestinal tract before they can be absorbed. The polysaccharide group includes starch and the undigestible carbohydrates that are commonly referred to as fiber.

The recommended intake of carbohydrate is 55 percent of the total daily energy intake. In an 8400 kJ (2000 kcal) diet this would be 275 g of carbohydrate, since each gram produces 16 kJ (4 kcal) of energy. The majority of the carbohydrate in one's diet should be obtained from complex carbohydrate rather than simple carbohydrate. Simple carbohydrates, such as refined sugars and concentrated sweets, contain energy but few other nutrients. For this reason, simple carbohydrates are often referred to as "empty-calorie" foods. This is not to say that they should not be included in the diet, but rather that they should be used in moderation as part of a well-balanced diet. The consumption of foods such as whole grain breads and cereals that contain complex carbohydrates is encouraged because these foods contain significant amounts of other nutrients. If energy needs are increased, as occurs with increased physical activity, desired weight gain, or during active IBD, the amount of carbohydrate included in the diet as a readily available energy source should also increase.

A deficiency of carbohydrate by itself is unusual. Most often, a carbohydrate deficiency occurs in association with a generally poor intake of all nutrients. This may arise during periods of acute active disease, when oral intake may be minimal. A carbohydrate deficiency leads to a loss of subcutaneous fat (the layer of fat just under the skin), muscle loss, a lack of energy, and weakness. If carbohydrate is lacking in the diet, the body will use protein or fat as an energy source. The use of protein as an energy source is wasteful because protein is expensive to buy and because the nitrogen (an essential constituent of protein foods) that would normally be used to build body proteins is excreted. If fat is used as the major energy source, breakdown products of fat metabolism can build up in the body to become a potential problem. For all of the these reasons, a diet lacking in carbohydrate is not encouraged.

Carbohydrate is generally well tolerated and absorbed by people with IBD. Active disease or surgical resection of the small intestine is usually not extensive enough to produce a carbohydrate deficiency through malabsorption. For some individuals, insufficient amounts of the lactose-splitting enzyme lactase in the digestive tract may result in the malabsorption of lactose. The inability to digest and absorb lactose is referred to as lactose intolerance. Although once thought to be more prevalent in individuals with IBD than in the general population, this is now known not to be true. If you are lactose intolerant, refer to the dietary modifications section for further information.

The major food sources of carbohydrate are the sugars and starches obtained from plant sources. Refined sugars, concentrated sweets, fruits, vegetables, nuts, and grains provide a variety of sugars and starches. Of animal-source foods, only those foods found in the milk group contain appreciable amounts of carbohydrate. Carbohydrate is not destroyed by cooking, but the type of carbohydrate available may be altered. For example, vegetables may become sweeter once cooked as disaccharides and polysaccharides are broken down to monosaccharides. Processing has the greatest effect on carbohydrates. For example, the refining of whole grains can result in significant losses of fiber, vitamins, and minerals because the bran layers and germ are removed during the refining process. As much as possible, a well-balanced diet based on the food guides is encouraged. Because most carbohydrate foods contain more than one nutrient, carbohydrate should be obtained from a variety of food sources to ensure a well-balanced intake of all nutrients. If you are required to modify your diet to reduce or increase the fiber content or to restrict lactose, refer to the appropriate sections listed in the dietary modifications section for further information. You are encouraged to discuss any concerns with your physician and registered dietitian before making any significant changes to your present diet.

MICRONUTRIENTS

Vitamins

Vitamins are a collection of unrelated compounds required by the body in very small amounts. They are grouped together because they are vital to many biological reactions within the body, are not a source of energy, are obtained from living matter, and can be readily altered or destroyed. Vitamins regulate metabolism, assist in the conversion of fat and carbohydrate into energy, and aid in the formation of bone and tissue. Most vitamins cannot be produced by the body, so they must be obtained from the diet. Vitamins are generally classified into two categories based on their solubility (capacity to dissolve). Vitamins dissolving in fat are referred to as fat-soluble vitamins; those dissolving in water are called water-soluble vitamins.

Fat-soluble vitamins: vitamin A, vitamin D, vitamin E, vitamin K

Water-soluble vitamins: B complex—thiamin (B_1), riboflavin (B_2), niacin (B_3), pyridoxine (B_6), folic acid, cobalamin (B_{12}), biotin, pantothenic acid; vitamin C

The following discussion will emphasize the situations that might promote the depletion of some of these vitamins in individuals with IBD. Keep in mind that vitamin deficiencies do not occur rapidly, but develop over time and are most often related to poor dietary habits superimposed on increased losses or needs. This information has been included to encourage you to follow a well-balanced diet at all times and to seek professional advice if you are not following a balanced diet.

It is hoped that you take an active role in your care and discuss any nutrition concerns you may have with your physician and registered dietitian.

FAT-SOLUBLE VITAMINS

Vitamin A

Vitamin A, the first fat-soluble vitamin to be recognized, is required for maintenance of healthy skin and inner mucous membranes, for normal resistance to infections, for bone and tooth development, and for normal vision. Vitamin A is absorbed in the upper portion of the small bowel in association with fat. As with all of the fat-soluble vitamins, any amount that is absorbed in excess of needs is stored in the body, particularly in the liver. The daily requirement for vitamin A for males and females between the ages of 19 and 24 is 1000 retinol equivalents (RE) and 800 RE, respectively, in both the United States and Canada. A deficiency of vitamin A in IBD patients can be related to one or a combination of the following: a diet unusually low in fat, fat malabsorption, or long-term use of the drug cholestyramine, which binds with fat-soluble vitamins, preventing their absorption. A deficiency of vitamin A may lead to changes in the skin and to night blindness (difficulty seeing in dim light).

Vitamin A is obtained from both plant and animal sources. Animal sources contain preformed vitamin A, whereas plant sources contain carotenes, which are converted to vitamin A in the body.

Sources of Vitamin A

Food Group	Food Sources	Comments
Milk group	Milk, cream, cheese	Good source of preformed vitamin A
Meat/alternate group	Beef liver and kidney, eggs	Liver an excellent source of preformed vitamin A
Bread/cereal group	No good sources	As a food group, a poor source
Fruit/vegetable group	Broccoli, spinach, pumpkin, winter squash, carrots, sweet potatoes, peaches, cantaloupe, dried apricots, mango, papayas	Carotene found in dark green or yellow-orange fruits and vegetables
Extra	Butter and fortified margarine	Can contribute to daily vitamin A intake

In general, vitamin A is relatively stable in most cooking methods. A well-balanced diet based on the food guides is more than adequate to meet most individuals' needs. Individuals on long-term cholestyramine therapy for bile-salt wasting or individuals with significant fat malabsorption may need vitamin A supplementation. Supplementation with vitamin A should only be undertaken on the advice of your physician and registered dietitian because vitamin A is stored in the liver, and an excessive intake may be hazardous.

Vitamin D

Vitamin D assists in the absorption and utilization of calcium, which is required for growth, development, and maintenance of healthy bones and teeth. Like vitamin A, dietary vitamin D is absorbed in the upper small bowel in conjunction with fats under the aid of bile salts. In addition to dietary intake, vitamin D can be formed in the body by the action of sunlight on skin. The recommended requirement for vitamin D in adult males and females aged 19 to 24 is 2.5 micrograms (μg) or 100 international units (IU) per day in Canada and quadruple that in the United States. An intake in excess of needs is stored in the liver, skin, and other tissues.

A deficiency state may develop in individuals with IBD as a result of a combination of factors such as a poor dietary intake, inadequate exposure to the sun, or fat malabsorption. A deficiency of vitamin D leads to osteomalacia and can lead to poor healing of bone fractures (break or rupture). Vitamin D is found in variable amounts in the fat of certain animal products, as listed in the table. Specific foods are regularly fortified with vitamin D and, when consumed daily, are often the major dietary source of this important nutrient.

Vitamin D is stable in ordinary cooking methods. With regular exposure to sunlight and a diet containing at least 250 mL (1 cup) of fortified milk per day,

Sources of Vitamin D

Food Group	Food Sources	Comments
Milk group	Fortified milk	Milk a good source because vitamin D is added to milk sold on the retail market
Meat/alternate group	Egg yolk, herring, salmon, canned sardines	Present in variable amounts in the fat of these foods
Bread/cereal group	No good sources	As a food group, a poor source
Fruit/vegetable group	No good sources	As a food group, a poor source
Extra	Butter, fortified margarine, fish liver oil	Fish liver oil is the best food source of vitamin D

vitamin D requirements will generally be met. Supplementation may be necessary for those individuals on long-term cholestyramine therapy, those with significant fat malabsorption, those who do not include milk in their diets, and those who have limited exposure to the sun. It is important to discuss any concerns you may have with your physician and registered dietitian. Supplementation of your diet with large amounts of vitamin D is to be avoided unless supervised by your physician because excessive amounts of this vitamin may produce toxic effects in bones and the liver.

Vitamin E

Vitamin E is often marketed to the general public as a substance to enhance sexual prowess and athletic ability as well as delay the aging process. In reality, the role of this vitamin is as an antioxidant (an agent that binds with oxygen to prevent unwanted changes). In this role, it protects vitamin A and polyunsaturated fatty acids (PUFA) from being destroyed, helps to maintain the health of membranes, and aids in the prevention of red blood cell destruction. Like other fat soluble vitamins, vitamin E is absorbed in the small intestine with the help of bile salts and fat. Summarizing the RNI and RDA, the requirement for this nutrient for adult males and females between the ages of 19 and 24 is 10 mg and 8 mg, respectively. Because this vitamin protects PUFA, the actual requirement depends on the dietary intake of PUFA. Unlike the other fat-soluble vitamins, this nutrient is stored in the body's fatty tissues rather than in the liver.

A deficiency of vitamin E in adults is rare, as it is readily available from a wide range of foods. In Crohn's disease, a deficiency may occur if losses exceed intake. This situation may arise in individuals who have undergone significant small bowel resection resulting in limited fat absorption. The unabsorbed fat binds

Sources of Vitamin E

Food Group	Food Sources	Comments
Milk group	Milk fat	Contributes to intake
Meat/alternate group	Liver, beef, egg yolk, nuts such as walnuts and peanuts	Liver an excellent source
Bread/cereal group	Wheat germ, whole-grain breads and cereals	Wheat germ a rich source
Fruit/vegetable group	Lettuce and other greens	Contributes to intake
Extra	Vegetable oils such as soybean, corn, and cottonseed	Excellent source

with the vitamin E in food and makes it unavailable for absorption into the body. A vitamin E deficiency results in destruction of red blood cells and various skin disorders. When compared to other vitamins, vitamin E is the most widely available from common foodstuffs. Interestingly, foods that contain PUFA are also good sources of vitamin E, so the intake of one ensures the intake of the other.

Vitamin E is not destroyed by heat and is insoluble in water. These characteristics make it stable in most methods of cooking. Because it is widely distributed in foods, a well-balanced diet, as outlined by the food guides, will ensure an adequate intake. Individuals with significant fat malabsorption caused by extensive small intestinal resection may need supplementation. Consult your physician and registered dietitian before taking a vitamin E supplement. As with all fat-soluble vitamins, excess intake is stored in the body, and when it is consumed in large amounts, it may give rise to adverse effects. Of the fat-soluble vitamins, excessive vitamin E intake is thought to be the least toxic, but unwanted side effects such as headache and blurred vision have been documented.

Vitamin K

Vitamin K derives its name from the Danish word *koagulation* because it plays an important role in the development of proteins necessary for blood clotting. Vitamin K is absorbed in the upper section of the small bowel with the help of bile and pancreatic enzymes. This vitamin is unusual in that it can be formed by bacteria in the lower intestinal tract. There are, therefore, two sources of this vitamin, the diet and normal bowel bacteria. In the United States, the RDA for adult males and adult females is 70 μg and 60 μg, respectively. It is thought that up to 50 percent of an individual's need can be provided by bacterial production in the intestine. An excess intake of vitamin K is stored to some extent in the liver. A deficiency of vitamin K is not common but has been identified in individuals with significant fat malabsorption and in situations where the growth of vitamin K-producing bacteria has been suppressed by antibiotic use and inadequate dietary vitamin K intake.

Sources of Vitamin K

Food Group	Food Sources	Comments
Milk group	Cheese	As a food group, a limited source
Meat/alternate group	Beef liver, egg yolk	As a food group, a limited source
Bread/cereal group	Wheat bran	As a food group, a limited source
Fruit/vegetable group	Asparagus, broccoli, cabbage, lettuce, spinach	Green leafy vegetables an excellent source

Vitamin K is found in significant amounts in green leafy vegetables, as well as in the foods noted in the table.

As with most fat-soluble vitamins, vitamin K is relatively stable in ordinary methods of cooking. This nutrient is destroyed by light, so proper storage is suggested. Store vitamin K-rich vegetables away from the light, such as in the crisper drawer of the refrigerator. A vitamin K deficiency is rare, and well-balanced diets, as outlined in the food guides, are more than adequate to meet most individuals' nutrient needs. A supplement may be required for individuals with significant fat malabsorption. As with all vitamin supplements, it is important to discuss your concerns with your physician and registered dietitian instead of self-prescribing supplementation. If a supplement is required, it is important that you receive professional advice, since large doses of vitamin K are potentially dangerous.

WATER-SOLUBLE VITAMINS

Thiamin

Thiamin (vitamin B_1) is one of several water-soluble vitamins grouped together and referred to under the term *B complex*. These nutrients are so grouped because they are generally obtained from similar food sources and have closely related functions. Thiamin is required by the body to help release energy from carbohydrates, to help transmit nerve impulses, and to aid in the metabolism of alcohol. Thiamin is readily absorbed in the upper section of the small intestine. As with most water-soluble vitamins, an intake above immediate need results in rapid excretion (the elimination from the body) of excess vitamin in the urine. Because of its role in releasing energy from carbohydrate, the requirement for this nutrient is related to the dietary consumption of carbohydrate and general energy intake. The daily requirement for adult males and females between the ages of 19 and 24 is approximately 1.5 mg and 1.1 mg, respectively.

By itself, a thiamin deficiency is not common, but it may arise in association with general malnutrition. Individuals with IBD who are at greatest risk for developing a deficiency are those who are following an unusually restricted diet, either from choice or from inability to tolerate foods or fluids for a prolonged period of time. The latter may arise during active disease, when nausea, vomiting, or diarrhea occur. A thiamin deficiency affects the nervous system and can result in a number of nonspecific complaints such as muscular weakness, emotional instability, and mental confusion. Thiamin is readily available from a wide number of foods, as noted in the table at the top of page 29.

As with many water-soluble vitamins, losses of this nutrient can be great with cooking. As the temperature and length of heating increases, the amount of thiamin destroyed also increases. Excessive water used in cooking allows the thiamin to leach out of the food and to be lost when the water is discarded. Careful attention to food preparation in association with a well-balanced diet that includes both raw

Sources of Thiamin

Food Group	Food Sources	Comments
Milk group	No good sources	As a food group a limited source, but contributory if consumed regularly
Meat/alternate group	Pork, liver and other organ meats, poultry, fish, eggs, dried beans and peas, nuts	Pork a very rich common food source
Bread/cereal group	Whole-grain and enriched breads and cereals, wheat germ	Many products enriched with this nutrient; wheat germ particularly rich
Fruit/vegetable group	Dark green vegetables	As a food group, a limited source

and cooked foods will provide adequate thiamin to meet nutrient needs. Refer to the section on retaining nutritional value for further discussion. Excessive ingestion of this nutrient has not been shown to be toxic, but supplementation should not be initiated without the advice of your physician and registered dietitian.

Riboflavin

Riboflavin (vitamin B_2) is involved in the release of energy from carbohydrate, protein, and fats and is essential for normal growth, development, and healthy skin. This nutrient is readily absorbed in the upper section of the small intestine. The requirement for riboflavin is based on energy intake; the daily requirement for adults between the ages of 19 and 24 is 1.5 and 1.7 mg for males and 1.1 and 1.3 mg for females in Canada and the United States, respectively. Like many water-soluble vitamins, riboflavin is not stored to any great extent in the body, and excess intake is excreted in the urine. There are very limited reserves of this nutrient in the liver and kidney. Therefore, riboflavin must be provided in the diet on a regular basis. A deficiency of this nutrient can result in cracked skin around the mouth and soreness or burning of the lips, tongue, and mouth. Burning and itching of the eyes and light sensitivity are other symptoms of deficiency. On its own, a riboflavin deficiency is rare, but IBD patients may develop it in association with general malnutrition if their diets are restricted for an extended period of time. Such a situation may occur with chronic active disease when associated with a poor diet.

This nutrient is found in many animal and vegetable foods but in small amounts.

Sources of Riboflavin

Food Group	Food Sources	Comments
Milk group	Milk, cheddar cheese, cottage cheese	Generally, foods high in calcium are a good source
Meat/alternate group	Organ meats, poultry, eggs	Organ meats especially high in riboflavin
Bread/cereal group	Enriched breads and cereals	Contributes to the daily intake
Fruit/vegetable group	Green leafy vegetables	Contributes to intake

This nutrient is very stable in usual methods of cooking because it is not affected by heat and has a limited solubility in water. Riboflavin is, however, sensitive to light, so foods should be stored in containers that protect against light. Sun-drying fruits and vegetables will result in some loss of this nutrient. Riboflavin is also sensitive to alkaline substances such as baking soda, and the practice of adding this powder to speed cooking and to enhance the color of vegetables is not encouraged. Refer to the section on retaining nutritional value for further discussion. A well-balanced diet as outlined by the food guide will provide more than adequate riboflavin to meet needs. To date, no toxic effects have been noted with excessive intake.

Niacin

Niacin (vitamin B_3) is involved in the release of energy from carbohydrate, protein, and fat. It is absorbed in the small intestine and is required on a regular basis, since body stores are limited. Niacin is unique because it can also be synthesized in the body from the amino acid tryptophan. Since it is involved in energy release, the recommended intake of niacin is based on energy intake. Summarizing the RNI and RDA, the daily requirement for adult males and females between the ages of 19 and 24 is approximately 20 NE (niacin equivalents) and 15 NE, respectively. An intake in excess of needs is readily excreted in the urine. A deficiency of this nutrient results in weakness, inflammation of the skin following exposure to light, mental confusion, and a general lack of energy. A niacin deficiency by itself is rare, but it may arise in association with general malnutrition. IBD patients have a higher risk for niacin deficiency if they are following a very restrictive diet for a prolonged period of time, especially if losses are increased. Such a situation may occur in active disease when the symptoms of pain, nausea, vomiting, and diarrhea

Sources of Niacin

Food Group	Food Sources	Comments
Milk group	Milk	Food group is a limited source of niacin but an excellent source of tryptophan
Meat/alternate group	Organ meats, peanut butter, legumes, lean meat, poultry, fish, eggs	Rich source of niacin
Bread/cereal group	Enriched products	May be bound to other compounds, which lessens its availability
Fruit/vegetable group	No good sources	A limited source

result in minimal dietary intake and increased losses. Niacin is easily obtained from a well-balanced diet.

Niacin is very stable in most common methods of cooking, although there are small losses in cooking water. A well-balanced diet based on the food guides will meet most individuals' needs. The ingestion of large doses of supplemental niacin have been associated with side effects, such as tingling sensations and flushing of the skin. Always discuss the use of large doses of any nutrient with your physician and registered dietitian.

Folacin (Folic Acid)

This vitamin is required for the formation and maturation of both red and white blood cells in the bone marrow. Folic acid is important in cell growth and re-production as well as the cellular utilization of proteins. It is absorbed from the upper section of the small bowel but can also be absorbed from the entire length of the small intestine. Summarizing the RNI and RDA, the daily recommended intake for folic acid for adult males and females between the ages of 19 and 24 is approximately 200 μg and 180 μg, respectively. As with all water-soluble vitamins, any intake in excess of needs is excreted in the urine.

Low concentrations of folic acid have been noted in individuals with IBD and are thought to be caused by one or several of the following factors: an increased requirement of the vitamin as a result of the rapid cell turnover of active disease; a decreased absorption caused by the interference by the drug sulfasalazine; an inadequate dietary intake, owing to poor eating habits or poor appetite; and overly restrictive diets without supplementation. Folic acid deficiency produces a type of anemia referred to as a megaloblastic anemia, which is characterized by red blood cells that are too large and too few in number. As a result, the oxygen-carrying ability of the blood is reduced.

The term *folacin* comes from the Latin word *folium*, meaning "leaf," because the vitamin is found in great concentrations in green leafy vegetables. Folic acid is also found in many other foods.

Significant amounts of folic acid can be lost during food processing, storage, and preparation. High temperatures, exposure to light, and the use of large volumes of cooking water can result in significant losses. Refer to the section on retaining nutritional value for further discussion. Even with losses, a well-balanced diet based on the food guides that includes whole grains and fresh dark green leafy vegetables will meet the needs of most individuals. Supplementation with folic acid should be discussed with your physician and registered dietitian when the drug sulfasalazine is used because it interferes with the absorption of folic acid. You should pay particular attention to the food sources of folic acid when you follow a restricted-fiber diet. If the diet is very restrictive and followed for a prolonged period of time, folic acid intake can be minimal since folic acid–rich foods are often omitted in restricted fiber diets. Folic acid supplementation should never be initiated without the knowledge of your physician because such supplementation may mask the signs of a vitamin B_{12} deficiency. Always discuss your concerns with your physician and registered dietitian before self-prescribing large supplemental doses of nutrients.

Sources of Folic Acid

Food Group	Food Sources	Comments
Milk group	No good sources	As a food group, a poor source
Meat/alternate group	Liver, nuts, seeds, red kidney beans, lima beans, soybeans	Liver, especially chicken liver, an excellent source
Bread/cereal group	Whole-wheat bread, whole-wheat flour, soy flour, bran cereals	Can be a good source if eaten regularly
Fruit/vegetable group	Brussels sprouts, spinach, asparagus, broccoli, beets, romaine lettuce, bean sprouts, parsnips, cauliflower, cantaloupe, oranges, orange juice	Fresh dark green leafy vegetables an excellent source

Vitamin B₁₂ (Cobalamin)

Vitamin B_{12} is required for normal red blood cell formation, for the maintenance of healthy nervous system tissue, and for normal gastrointestinal function. Unlike most other vitamins, vitamin B_{12} is absorbed specifically in the terminal ileum. This nutrient is also unique among the water-soluble vitamins because it is stored extensively in the body, with reserves often adequate for 2 to 7 years following interference with absorption. The recommended intake for B_{12} for both adult males and females is 2 μg per day in the United States and 1 μg per day in Canada.

A deficiency of vitamin B_{12} in individuals with IBD may result from prolonged inadequate dietary intake. However, this is rare in people who are not vegans (strict vegetarians who consume no foods from an animal source). Deficiency is more frequently caused by removal of or damage to the terminal ileum. In Crohn's disease, surgical removal of all or part of the ileum, extensive chronic ileal disease, or bacterial overgrowth in the ileum may contribute to a vitamin B_{12} deficiency. A B_{12} deficiency results in megaloblastic anemia and changes to the nervous system that, if not detected and treated, may be irreversible. The ingestion of large amounts of folic acid in the presence of a vitamin B_{12} deficiency may correct the megaloblastic anemia but will not prevent the progressive nerve damage. A very simple blood test will detect a vitamin B_{12} deficiency. It is recommended that vitamin B_{12} status be checked regularly in any individual at risk for depletion.

Vitamin B_{12} is widely available in foods of animal origin. Foods of plant origin are devoid of this nutrient, with the exception of bacterially fermented soy products.

Vitamin B_{12} is relatively heat-stable, and losses in cooking are not as significant as with other water-soluble vitamins. If a deficiency is present, regular monthly injections of vitamin B_{12} will be required to correct the deficiency. Oral supplements of vitamin B_{12} will not be absorbed if the underlying problem is

Sources of Vitamin B_{12}

Food Group	Food Sources	Comments
Milk group	Milk, cheese	Good source
Meat/alternate group	Beef liver, kidney, heart, clams, oysters, eggs, fermented soybean foods	Liver and kidney an excellent source
Bread/cereal group	No good sources	As a food group, a poor source
Fruit/vegetable group	No good sources	A poor source

malabsorption related to disease or resection of the ileum. No toxic effects of excessive supplementation have been documented. Because animal products are the main food source of vitamin B_{12}, individuals who follow a very strict vegetarian diet, such as vegans, are at significant risk for developing a deficiency of this important nutrient. It is highly recommended that strict vegetarians seek further advice from a registered dietitian.

Pyridoxine

Pyridoxine (vitamin B_6) is involved in protein synthesis, the production of anti-bodies and red blood cells, and the normal functioning of the nervous system. Like many of the water-soluble vitamins, pyridoxine is absorbed in the upper small intestine. Because of its relationship to protein utilization, the requirement for pyridoxine is based on protein intake. For adult men and women between the ages of 19 and 24, the recommended daily intake in the United States is approximately 2 mg and 1.6 mg, respectively. Any intake in excess of need is excreted in the urine; body stores are therefore limited.

By itself, a pyridoxine deficiency is uncommon. However, a deficiency may develop in individuals with IBD as part of general malnutrition. Such a situation may arise if illness interferes with the consumption of a balanced diet over a prolonged period of time. A deficiency of pyridoxine may cause dizziness, convulsions, and behavior changes. Pyridoxine is found in many foods of both plant and animal origin, and a good intake is easily achieved when following a balanced diet.

Pyridoxine is unstable in light, and, as a water-soluble nutrient, losses can be great with food storage, preparation, and cooking. Refer to the section on retaining nutritional value for information on reducing nutrient loss from foods. The use of large supplemental doses of pyridoxine can result in dizziness and seizures. Always discuss the use of supplements with your physician and registered dietitian.

Sources of Pyridoxine

Food Group	Food Sources	Comments
Milk group	Milk	Generally a limited source
Meat/alternate group	Meat, liver, dried beans and peas, nuts	Liver an especially good source
Bread/cereal group	Whole-grain cereals	Contributes to intake
Fruit/vegetable group	Dark green leafy vegetables, potatoes	As a group, a limited source

Vitamin C

Vitamin C is required for the production of collagen, a protein substance found in all fibrous tissue including connective tissue, cartilage, and skin. In this role, vitamin C preserves capillary strength (capillaries are tiny, thin-walled blood vessels that connect the smallest arteries with the smallest veins), which promotes the healing of wounds and reduces the risk of infections. Vitamin C also aids in the absorption of iron. This nutrient is readily absorbed from the upper section of the small intestine. In the United States, the RDA for this nutrient for adult males and females is 60 mg. In Canada, the RNI is 40 mg for men and 30 mg for women, with the recommendation that smokers increase vitamin C intake by 50 percent. An intake in excess of needs is excreted in the urine.

Vitamin C deficiency has been noted in individuals with IBD and is thought to be caused by a poor dietary intake from overly restrictive low-fiber diets. In addition, increased losses through diarrhea and increased needs for healing may contribute. A deficiency, especially in active IBD, is thought to delay wound healing and reduce resistance to infections.

Almost all of the daily intake of vitamin C is obtained from fruits and vegetables. Generally, vitamin C is found in highest concentrations in food fresh from the plant. For this reason, vitamin C has been referred to as the "fresh-food vitamin."

Vitamin C is easily destroyed by air, light, and heat. Therefore, the amount of vitamin C available in a food depends heavily on proper storage and preparation. Raw fruits and vegetables and their juices are preferred to cooked items whenever possible. Refer to the section on retaining nutritional value for further discussion. If a restricted-fiber diet is necessary, it is important to make wise food choices to ensure that vitamin C intake meets one's needs. Cantaloupe and honeydew melon are foods that are lower in fiber but are good sources of vitamin C. Fruit juices such as orange and grapefruit juice are low in fiber and are encouraged as a source of this important nutrient.

Sources of Vitamin C

Food Group	Food Sources	Comments
Milk group	No good sources	Poor source
Meat/alternate group	No good sources	Poor source
Bread/cereal group	No good sources	Poor source
Fruit/vegetable group	Oranges, grapefruits, their juices, kiwi fruit, cantaloupe, strawberries, tomato juice, broccoli, spinach	Citrus fruits and raw leafy greens are excellent sources

If vitamin C–rich foods are taken, supplementation with vitamin C is usually not required, even if a restricted-fiber diet is followed. For example, one orange or 125 mL ($\frac{1}{2}$ cup) orange juice contains 60 to 65 mg of vitamin C, which meets one day's requirement. Large doses of supplemental vitamin C are discouraged, as nausea, abdominal cramps, and diarrhea have been reported with excessive intakes. In addition, consuming large amounts of vitamin C on a regular basis has been associated with kidney stone formation. Always consult your physician and registered dietitian before taking large doses of nutrients.

Minerals

In nutrition, the term *mineral* refers to an inorganic element (one that does not contain carbon) that is in its simplest form and cannot be broken down or destroyed. As inorganic substances, minerals are present in earth rather than originating from living matter. Minerals have many essential roles. They regulate the metabolism of many enzymes, maintain proper nerve and muscle function, and are indirectly involved in the growth process. Like vitamins, minerals are required by the body in small amounts. Minerals can be subdivided into two groups depending on the amount in the body. Minerals found in the body in relatively large amounts are referred to as major minerals, and those found in the body in relatively small amounts are referred to as trace minerals.

> *Major minerals:* calcium, phosphorous, sodium, potassium, chlorine, magnesium, sulfur
>
> *Trace minerals:* iron, iodine, zinc, copper, manganese, cobalt, fluorine, selenium, chromium, molybdenum.

Of the essential minerals, only those of greatest interest to individuals with IBD will be discussed. As with the section on vitamins, this information is presented to encourage you to follow a well-balanced diet and to contact your physician and registered dietitian with any concerns.

CALCIUM

Calcium is required for the formation and maintenance of strong bones and teeth, maintenance of muscle tone and normal heart beat, proper blood clotting, and healthy nerve function. This nutrient is absorbed in the duodenum (the first portion of the small intestine), but may be absorbed to a lesser extent in other areas of the intestine. In the United States, the RDA is 1200 mg for adult males and females between the ages of 19 and 24. In Canada, the RNI is 700 mg for adult females and 800 mg for adult males. An intake in excess of needs is not absorbed from the intestinal tract. Bone acts as a reservoir for calcium and will release the mineral to maintain normal blood levels.

There is a high risk for calcium depletion in individuals with IBD; this may contribute to bone diseases such as osteomalacia and osteoporosis. Factors that contribute to calcium depletion include a deficiency of vitamin D, which is required for calcium absorption; calcium malabsorption resulting from steatorrhea or diarrhea; and reduced calcium absorption resulting from interference by the drug prednisone. Calcium stores may also be reduced as a direct result of a poor dietary intake because of a true or presumed lactose intolerance. You are encouraged to refer to the dietary modifications section for further information on lactose intolerance.

Calcium can be obtained from certain breads and cereals as well as fruits and vegetables, but binders such as phytic acid and oxalic acid in these foods render the calcium relatively unavailable. However, some calcium is absorbed from these sources and contributes to the total daily intake. Milk and milk products are the best sources of calcium, and it is difficult to meet nutritional needs if the milk group is omitted.

Calcium is not affected by usual storage or preparation methods. Supplementation is not generally required because a well-balanced diet containing milk and milk products will meet most individuals' needs. Five hundred mL (2 cups) of milk

Sources of Calcium

Food Group	Food Sources	Comments
Milk group	All	Excellent source. In milk calcium absorption aided by added vitamin D
Meat/alternate group	Sardines and salmon with bones, clams, oysters, cheese, cottage cheese, tofu, almonds, dry beans, chick peas	Fish bones an excellent source
Bread/cereal group	Bran cereals, oatmeal, carob flour, soybean flour, baked goods containing added dried milk solids and/or added calcium carbonate	Calcium less well absorbed because it is bound with phytic acid
Fruit/vegetable group	Broccoli, spinach, swiss chard, rhubarb	Calcium from these foods less well absorbed because it is bound with oxalic acid

combined with 30 g (1 oz) of cheese provides 800 mg of calcium. When needs are increased, as in prolonged use of prednisone, increasing the daily intake of foods from the milk group to twice the recommended amount often meets requirements. Refer to the section on dietary modifications for further information on how to improve the calcium content of your diet. A very high intake of calcium in the presence of a high intake of vitamin D, such as may occur in individuals taking potent commercial supplements, is a potential source of elevated blood calcium levels. This may lead to the unwanted deposition of calcium in soft tissues such as the kidneys. Supplementation with calcium and vitamin D should always be discussed with your physician and registered dietitian.

SODIUM

Because sodium is so readily available in our diet, it is easy to forget that sodium is an important nutrient required by the body on a regular basis. Sodium is an indispensable body component that is found distributed in both body fluids and tissue. It is required for the maintenance of normal water balance, nerve conduction, and muscle function. Sodium is readily absorbed from the gastrointestinal tract in both the small and large intestine. In North America, daily intakes of sodium often far exceed the suggested reasonable intake of approximately 3 g per day. It is estimated that the average North American diet provides more than 6 g of sodium per day. Sodium requirements increase when losses are greater, such as those occurring with heavy sweating, diarrhea, and vomiting. Generally, the greater the intake of sodium, the greater the amount absorbed. A state of balance is maintained through the rapid excretion in the urine of the excess intake. When sodium concentrations in the blood rise too high, thirst is stimulated and one drinks more fluid. When blood concentration of sodium is too low, losses in the urine decrease. In IBD, a sodium deficiency may arise when oral intake is inadequate or if losses are increased because of vomiting or diarrhea. A sodium deficiency results in muscle weakness and confusion. Normally, a deficiency of sodium is rare, as this mineral is found in a wide range of foods. The amount of sodium available from natural sources is limited when compared to the amount available in processed foods such as ham, luncheon meats, condiments such as soy sauce, and snack foods such as potato chips. Adding sodium in the form of sodium chloride (table salt) to foods is a significant source of sodium.

Individuals with IBD experiencing diarrhea and vomiting should consume foods and fluids that are rich in sodium. Refer to the dietary modifications section for further information on diarrhea. Individuals who have ileostomies (a surgically created opening through the abdominal wall into the ileum) may have an increased requirement for sodium, owing to increased losses. Unless advised by your physician, sodium intake should not be restricted. However, because sodium aggravates high blood pressure, it is wise to reduce sodium intake if you have been diagnosed with this medical problem. It is recommended that you seek further advice from your physician and registered dietitian.

POTASSIUM

Potassium is involved in the release of energy, protein synthesis, maintenance of normal water balance, and neuromuscular activity. This important mineral is readily absorbed from the small intestine. There is no recommended intake for potassium, but a suggested safe and adequate daily intake for adults is estimated between 1.9 and 5.6 grams per day. An excess intake is readily excreted in the urine.

Potassium deficiency in IBD patients may result from prolonged inadequate dietary intake. More commonly, a deficiency results from chronic diarrhea or vomiting, which increase losses. In diarrhea, the passage of intestinal contents is so rapid that there is a decreased absorption of dietary potassium and an increased loss of potassium in the digestive secretions that are not absorbed. The chief symptoms of potassium deficiency are muscular weakness, rapid heart rate, and mental confusion.

Potassium is readily available from a wide variety of foods.

Although indestructible, minerals such as potassium can be readily leached out of food resulting in considerable amounts being lost in cooking water. In order to retain as much potassium as possible, raw fruits and vegetables or their juices should be eaten. When cooking foods, use as little water as possible, and cook for the shortest amount of time. Refer to the section on retaining nutritional value for

Sources of Potassium

Food Group	Food Sources	Comments
Milk group	Milk, including powdered skim milk	Rich in potassium
Meat/alternate group	Scallops, sardines, calves' liver, lima beans, peanuts, soybeans	Rich in potassium
Bread/cereal group	Bran cereals	As a food group, a poor source
Fruit/vegetable group	Dried apricots, melon, citrus fruits, bananas, dates, potatoes, mushrooms, parsnips, spinach, squash, broccoli, brussels sprouts	Excellent source

further information. In IBD, potassium supplementation is usually only required when dietary intake is poor and diarrhea, vomiting, or both are present. When diarrhea is present, such as may occur in active disease, it is most important that a potassium-rich diet is consumed. The easiest way to achieve this goal is to drink citrus juices daily, which will not only replace potassium but also provide fluid. Because potassium is water soluble, dietary intake in excess of needs is rapidly excreted in the urine, and toxicity is not generally a concern unless kidney failure is present. However, like any supplement, potassium supplements should be used only on the advice of your physician, since an excessive intake can be hazardous.

MAGNESIUM

Magnesium is essential for the normal functioning of muscle and nerve tissue, the utilization of carbohydrate and protein, and the formation and maintenance of bone. This mineral is absorbed along the entire length of the small intestine. In Canada, the RNI for adult males and females between the ages of 19 and 24 is 240 mg and 200 mg, respectively. In the United States, the RDA is slightly higher at 350 mg for adult males and 280 mg for adult females. A magnesium deficiency may develop in individuals with IBD who are experiencing ongoing diarrhea as a result of active disease or significant small bowel resection and who are consuming a poor diet. In addition, the risk of magnesium deficiency increases in individuals experiencing steatorrhea or those consuming large amounts of calcium supplements. Unabsorbed fats in the small intestine bind magnesium and make it unavailable for absorption. Large amounts of calcium interfere with the absorption of magnesium by competing for absorption. A magnesium deficiency results in depression, muscular weakness, dizziness, and convulsions.

Sources of Magnesium

Food Group	Food Sources	Comments
Milk group	Milk	A poor source
Meat/alternate group	Shrimp, clams, oysters, prawns, sardines, salmon, nuts and nut butters, dried peas and beans	Seafood a good source
Bread/cereals group	Whole-grain flour, bread, cereals	A good source
Fruit/vegetable group	Dried fruits, spinach, potatoes, beans, cabbage	Dark green leafy vegetables an especially good source

Magnesium occurs abundantly in foods, and a well-balanced diet based on the food guides with an inclusion of whole grains and dark green leafy vegetables meets the needs of most individuals.

Dietary magnesium is very water soluble, so considerable amounts may be lost in cooking water. In order to retain as much magnesium in foods as possible, use cooking methods that use little water, and cook for the shortest time. For individuals who have had a significant amount of the small intestine removed, magnesium supplements may be necessary. Individuals who are following strict fiber-restricted diets over an extended period of time may also require supplementation. It is important not to take large amounts of supplemental magnesium unless directed by your physician and registered dietitian because oral magnesium supplementation may cause diarrhea and upset stomach.

IRON

Iron is present in every cell of the body, with the majority being found in the red blood cells as part of hemoglobin. Hemoglobin is responsible for the transport of oxygen from the lungs to the body tissues. Iron also plays a role in maintaining immune function and resistance to infections. Iron is absorbed in the upper small intestine, with about 10 percent of dietary intake being absorbed. In the United States, the RDA for adult males and females between the ages of 19 and 24 is 10 mg and 15 mg, respectively. In Canada, the RNI is 9 mg for men and 13 mg for women.

Iron deficiency may result in anemia (a reduction in hemoglobin or an insufficient number of red blood cells). When the anemia is caused by a deficiency of iron, the red blood cells contain little hemoglobin and carry less oxygen. The classic symptom of iron deficiency anemia is a constant feeling of weariness. Anemia tends to be a common nutritional deficiency in the general population, particularly in women; this is thought to be caused in part by an inadequate dietary intake superimposed on regular losses with menstruation. Anemia from iron deficiency is also common in IBD and is thought to be caused by chronic blood loss from the gastrointestinal tract and poor dietary intake. In addition, fat malabsorption and diarrhea may interfere with iron absorption. Another cause of insufficient iron in IBD is a defective release of iron into the blood from body iron stores. This is not a true iron deficiency, but inadequate utilization of body iron stores, owing to the disease process.

There are two forms of dietary iron: heme-iron and non-heme-iron. Heme-iron is found in animal-source foods, such as meat, fish, and poultry. It is much better absorbed than non-heme-iron, which is found in plant-source foods such as fruits, vegetables, and grains. The absorption of non-heme-iron is improved greatly by vitamin C. Therefore, drinking orange juice or eating any food high in vitamin C

Sources of Iron

Food Group	Food Sources	Comments
Milk group	No good sources	As a group, a poor source
Meat/alternate group	Liver, kidney, heart, beef, pork, lamb, oysters, clams, sardines, shrimp, lentils, dried beans, peas	Organ meats an excellent source of heme-iron; dried beans, peas, and lentils a good source of non-heme-iron
Bread/cereal group	Whole grains and enriched breads and cereals	A good source of non-heme-iron
Fruit/vegetable group	Raisins, dried apricots, dried peaches, spinach	A good source of non-heme-iron

with a meal is encouraged. In addition, the absorption of non-heme-iron is enhanced by the presence of heme-iron. Choosing both heme- and non-heme-iron-containing foods at a meal improves iron absorption.

Iron is relatively stable in most methods of storage, preparation, and cooking. Cooking can actually enhance the amount of iron obtained from the diet, since preparation in iron pans will add iron to the food. Scrambling eggs in an iron frying pan can double or triple the iron content. Individuals with IBD, especially women with regular monthly menstrual losses, should consume an iron-rich diet. Refer to the section on dietary modifications for advice on improving iron intake. Sometimes even with a well-balanced diet, iron supplementation may be necessary. Iron supplementation should only be undertaken upon the advice of a physician because an excessive intake can result in liver damage. Since it is more difficult to meet iron needs when following a vegetarian diet, individuals following such a diet are encouraged to consult their physician and registered dietitian for more detailed advice.

ZINC

Zinc plays a role in many vital enzyme systems involved in energy and protein metabolism. This nutrient is required for wound healing, maintenance of healthy tissues, and normal sense of taste. Zinc is absorbed in the upper small intestine. In the United States, the requirement for this nutrient is 15 mg for adult males and 12 mg for adult females. In Canada, the zinc requirement for an adult male and an adult female is 12 mg and 9 mg per day, respectively. A zinc deficiency may lead

Sources of Zinc

Food Group	Food Sources	Comments
Milk group	Dry nonfat milk	As a group, a limited source
Meat/alternate group	Beef, lamb, liver, pork, turkey, shellfish, oysters, egg yolk, dried beans	Good source, especially seafood
Bread/cereal group	Whole-grain breads and cereals, wheat germ	Can be a good source, but zinc not readily absorbed because of fiber and phytic acid
Fruit/vegetable group	Corn, beets, peas	As a group, a limited source

to hair loss, loss of taste and smell, and growth retardation. In individuals with IBD, a zinc deficiency may develop as a consequence of prolonged restricted dietary intake associated with poor appetite or poor food choices, impaired absorption caused by diarrhea, and increased requirements during active disease.

Animal foods are good sources of zinc. Cereal grains, although rich in zinc, contain fiber and phytic acid, which interfere with zinc absorption.

Zinc is a very stable nutrient, with minimal loss in cooking, storage, and preparation. A well-balanced diet based on the food guides that emphasizes whole grains and includes two servings of animal protein per day will meet most individuals' needs. Individuals who follow a diet that omits all animal protein should seek advice from their physician and registered dietitian. Some situations, such as a period of acute active disease with significant diarrhea and poor intake, may require the use of a supplement. Supplementation with large doses of zinc should only be initiated on the advice of your physician and registered dietitian, since an excessive intake may interfere with iron and copper balance.

RETAINING THE NUTRITIONAL VALUE OF FOOD

Good nutrition is essential to good health in individuals with IBD. Wise daily food choices based on the food guides help to ensure a well-balanced intake of the essential nutrients. It is most important once foods are purchased that they be properly handled in order to retain as much of their nutritional value as possible.

Although many individuals feel that industrial processing is the main contributor to nutrient loss from foods, the major offenders are improper storage and preparation of food prior to consumption. Loss of vitamins and minerals from plant sources is the greatest concern. The following are the most common contributors to nutrient loss from fresh produce:

- Spoilage
- Excessive processing, peeling, cutting, slicing, washing, soaking
- Unnecessarily large amounts of water in cooking
- Excessive use of heat in cooking
- Discarding of cooking water
- Storing of cooked foods for longer than 1 to 2 days
- Reheating

GUIDELINES FOR MAXIMIZING THE NUTRIENT CONTENT OF FOODS

In order to ensure that you retain as much of the nutritional value of your food as possible, be aware of the following guidelines.

Selection

- Purchase only fresh fruits and vegetables that are free from excessive bruising and wilting in order to minimize the loss of vitamins A and C.

Storage

- Once purchased, store produce properly and as quickly as possible.
- Store vegetables in a plastic bag or in a crisper in the refrigerator.
- Store tube or root vegetables, such as potatoes, onions, or squash, in a cool, well-ventilated place.
- Store cut fruit and vegetables in the refrigerator in a covered container to retain vitamin C content.

Preparation

- Eat fresh, raw fruits and vegetables rather than cooked produce as much as possible.
- Prepare vegetables immediately before cooking and serving.
- During preparation, do not bruise produce, as this exposes cellular contents to air and reduces the content of vitamins A and C.
- Scrub, but do not peel, vegetables.

(Continued)

(Continued)
- To retain water-soluble nutrients, refrain from cutting vegetables into small pieces to cook.
- Try to avoid soaking vegetables, but if you must, soak with the peel intact to reduce loss of water-soluble nutrients.

Cooking

- Cook vegetables in their skins whenever possible.
- When boiling vegetables, boil the water before adding the vegetables and return to boiling as soon as possible in order to reduce loss of vitamin C and thiamin.
- When boiling foods, use as little water as possible in a tight fitting pot and minimize the cooking time.
- Save the cooking water and use it as stock in soups and gravies. The water is very rich in water-soluble nutrients.
- Never use baking soda when cooking vegetables because this will destroy thiamin and vitamin C.
- Better methods of cooking vegetables than boiling are microwaving, steaming, sautéing, stir frying, and pressure cooking if little water is used and cooking time is short.
- Deep fat frying of vegetables reduces the amount of many heat-sensitive vitamins. Therefore, avoid this method of cooking when possible.
- Cooked vegetables lose some nutrients in storage, and reheating results in further nutrient loss. Try to cook only the amount of vegetables that you need for a single meal to reduce leftovers.

3

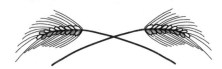

Dietary Modifications

A well-balanced diet as outlined by the food guides should be followed by all individuals with IBD. However, certain situations may necessitate a temporary or permanent alteration to the usual diet. This may be in the form of a texture modification, food or nutrient restriction, or food or nutrient inclusion. As dietary modifications carry the potential for a nutritionally unbalanced intake, the advice of a registered dietitian is encouraged. This guidance is particularly important if the dietary modification is to be long term.

The following pages address some common dietary modifications that individuals with IBD may be requested to follow. Included is information on the rationale for the dietary modification, general dietary guidelines, sample menus, and advice on improving the nutritional value of the diet. This information is not intended to replace professional nutritional advice, but to provide supplemental guidance only.

CLEAR FLUID DIET

Minimal stool production and intestinal activity result when a clear fluid diet is consumed. This diet is often used for a short period during acute active disease, following surgery, or in preparation for diagnostic tests. Because it allows only clear, nonspiced fluids or foods that liquify soon after eating, this diet is nutritionally inadequate and should not be the sole source of nutrition if used for longer than two days. Various commercial nutritional supplements are available that can be added to the clear fluid diet to markedly improve its nutritional value. A balanced multivitamin and mineral supplement should be taken if a clear fluid diet is required for more than two days.

FOODS ALLOWED

- Clear broth, bouillon, consommé
- Water, ice, clear tea, coffee
- Clear fruit juices and fruit drinks such as apple juice, Tang™, Kool-Aid™

Sample Clear Fluid Diet

Meal	Food Item	Amount	Energy kJ	Energy kcal	Protein (g)
Breakfast	Apple juice	250 mL (1 cup)	525	125	1
	Tea	250 mL (1 cup)	0	0	0
Lunch	Orange juice	250 mL (1 cup)	460	110	2
	Beef broth	250 mL (1 cup)	42	10	1
	Cherry gelatin	125 mL ($\frac{1}{2}$ cup)	315	75	2
	Tea	250 mL (1 cup)	0	0	0
Snack	Grape juice	250 mL (1 cup)	695	165	1
Evening meal	Apple juice	250 mL (1 cup)	525	125	1
	Chicken broth	250 mL (1 cup)	42	10	1
	Orange gelatin	250 mL (1 cup)	630	150	4
	Tea	250 mL (1 cup)	0	0	0
Snack	Popsicle	1	250	60	0
Total			3485	830	13

- Popsicles™
- Clear flavored gelatin
- Clear carbonated beverages such as ginger-ale and lemon-lime-flavored soda
- Sugar, honey, clear hard candies
- Herbs and mild seasonings such as salt and flavor extracts
- Some commercial supplements (refer to the section on commercial supplements)

Sample High-Energy High-Protein Clear Fluid Diet

Meal	Food Item	Amount	Energy kJ	Energy kcal	Protein (g)
Breakfast	Apple juice with	250 mL (1 cup)	525	125	1
	Polycose®*	30 mL (2 tbsp)	250	60	0
	Tea with	250 mL (1 cup)	0	0	0
	Honey	15 mL (1 tbsp)	275	65	0
Snack	Citrotein®*	250 mL (1 cup)	715	170	10.5
Lunch	Orange juice with	250 mL (1 cup)	460	110	2
	Polycose*	30 mL (2 tbsp)	250	60	0
	Beef consommé	250 mL (1 cup)	125	30	4
	Cherry gelatin made	250 mL (1 cup)	630	150	4
	with Polycose*	30 mL (2 tbsp)	250	60	0
	Tea with	250 mL (1 cup)	0	0	0
	Honey	15 mL (1 tbsp)	275	65	0
Snack	Citrotein*	250 mL (1 cup)	715	170	10.5
Evening meal	Apple juice with	250 mL (1 cup)	525	125	1
	Polycose*	30 mL (2 tbsp)	250	60	0
	Beef consommé	250 mL (1 cup)	128	30	4
	Orange gelatin with	250 mL (1 cup)	630	150	4
	Polycose*	30 mL (2 tbsp)	250	60	0
	Tea with	250 mL (1 cup)	0	0	0
	Honey	15 mL (1 tbsp)	275	65	0
Snack	Citrotein*	250 mL (1 cup)	715	170	10.5
Total			7240	1725	51.5

* Or equivalent. Refer to section on commercial supplements.

TIPS TO IMPROVE THE NUTRITIONAL VALUE OF THE CLEAR
FLUID DIET

- Make gelatin and popsicles with fruit juice, or clear carbonated beverages.
- Add extra sugar or honey to tea, juices, fruit drinks.
- Incorporate commercial supplements into the daily diet (as required).
- Take a well-balanced multivitamin and mineral supplement daily.

FULL FLUID DIET

To a lesser extent than clear fluids, this diet provides for some reduction in intestinal activity and stool production as compared to a solid diet. The full fluid diet

Sample Full Fluid Diet

Meal	Food Item	Amount	Energy		Protein (g)
			kJ	kcal	
Breakfast	Orange juice	250 mL (1 cup)	460	110	2
	2% milk	125 mL ($\frac{1}{2}$ cup)	275	65	4.5
	Strained oatmeal	125 mL ($\frac{1}{2}$ cup)	295	70	2
	with 2% milk	50 mL ($\frac{1}{4}$ cup)	135	32	2
	and Brown sugar	15 mL (1 tbsp)	140	34	0
Snack	Plain yogurt	125 mL ($\frac{1}{2}$ cup)	335	80	7
Lunch	Apple juice	125 mL ($\frac{1}{2}$ cup)	250	60	0.5
	2% milk	250 mL (1 cup)	545	130	9
	Tomato soup made with				
	whole milk	250 mL (1 cup)	715	170	6
	Vanilla pudding	125 mL ($\frac{1}{2}$ cup)	840	200	3
Snack	Orange sherbet	125 mL ($\frac{1}{2}$ cup)	610	145	1
Evening meal	Tomato juice	125 mL ($\frac{1}{2}$ cup)	85	20	1
	2% milk	250 mL (1 cup)	545	130	9
	Strained cream of				
	mushroom soup made				
	with whole milk	250 mL (1 cup)	905	215	6
	Vanilla ice cream	125 mL ($\frac{1}{2}$ cup)	590	140	3
Snack	Baked custard	125 mL ($\frac{1}{2}$ cup)	670	160	8
Total			7395	1760	64

is often used as a transition from clear fluids to solids during active disease or following intestinal surgery. Unlike clear fluids, a full fluid diet is more nutritionally complete, palatable, and satisfying. To ensure a balanced intake of all nutrients, a multivitamin and mineral supplement should be considered if this diet is to be used for more than three to five days. If you have a lactose intolerance, this diet will

Sample High-Energy High-Protein Full Fluid Diet

Meal	Food Item	Amount	Energy kJ	Energy kcal	Protein (g)
Breakfast	Orange juice with	125 mL ($\frac{1}{2}$ cup)	230	55	1
	Polycose*	15 mL (1 tbsp)	125	30	0
	Enriched milk†	250 mL (1 cup)	1155	275	20
	Strained oatmeal with	125 mL ($\frac{1}{2}$ cup)	295	70	2
	Cream and	50 mL ($\frac{1}{4}$ cup)	360	86	2
	Brown sugar	15 mL (1 tbsp)	140	34	0
Snack	Enriched milk†	250 mL (1 cup)	1155	275	20
Lunch	Apple juice with	125 mL ($\frac{1}{2}$ cup)	250	60	0.5
	Polycose*	15 mL (1 tbsp)	125	30	0
	Enriched milk†	250 mL (1 cup)	1155	275	20
	Tomato soup made				
	with Whole milk	250 mL (1 cup)	715	170	6
	and Butter	15 mL (1 tbsp)	420	100	0
	Vanilla pudding	125 mL ($\frac{1}{2}$ cup)	840	200	3
Snack	Vanilla shake†	1 serving	1825	435	20
Evening meal	Tomato juice	125 mL ($\frac{1}{2}$ cup)	85	20	1
	Enriched milk†	250 mL (1 cup)	1155	275	20
	Strained cream of mushroom soup made				
	with Whole milk	250 mL (1 cup)	905	215	6
	and Butter	15 mL (1 tbsp)	420	100	0
	Vanilla ice cream	125 mL ($\frac{1}{2}$ cup)	590	140	3
Snack	Baked custard	125 mL ($\frac{1}{2}$ cup)	670	160	8
Total			12615	3005	132.5

* Or equivalent. Refer to the section on commercial supplements.

† Refer to recipe section.

require modification because milk is the major component of the foods allowed. This diet allows only low-fiber, non-spiced fluids or foods that liquify soon after being eaten.

FOODS ALLOWED

- Clear fluid diet items
- Milk and milk-based beverages such as milkshakes, Instant Breakfast™
- Plain and flavored yogurt (no solids)
- Puddings, custards, ice cream, plain sherbet
- Vegetable juice (no pulp)

Sample Restricted-Lactose Full Fluid Diet

Meal	Food Item	Amount	Energy		Protein (g)
			kJ	kcal	
Breakfast	Orange juice	125 mL ($\frac{1}{2}$ cup)	230	55	1
	Treated* 2% milk	250 mL (1 cup)	545	130	9
	Strained oatmeal with	125 mL ($\frac{1}{2}$ cup)	294	70	2
	Brown sugar	15 mL (1 tbsp)	140	34	0
	Tea with	250 mL (1 cup)	0	0	0
	Honey	15 mL (1 tbsp)	275	65	0
Snack	Treated* milk	125 mL ($\frac{1}{2}$ cup)	275	65	4.5
Lunch	Apple juice	125 mL ($\frac{1}{2}$ cup)	250	60	0.5
	Treated* 2% milk	250 mL (1 cup)	545	130	9
	Tomato soup made with Treated*				
	whole milk	250 mL (1 cup)	715	170	6
	Orange gelatin	125 mL ($\frac{1}{2}$ cup)	315	75	2
Snack	Treated* 2% milk	125 mL ($\frac{1}{2}$ cup)	275	65	4.5
Evening meal	Tomato juice	125 mL ($\frac{1}{2}$ cup)	85	20	1
	Treated* 2% milk	250 mL (1 cup)	545	130	9
	Strained beef soup	250 mL (1 cup)	170	40	4
	Lime gelatin	125 mL ($\frac{1}{2}$ cup)	315	75	2
Snack	Popsicle	1	250	60	0
Total			5225	1245	54.5

* Treated milk refers to milk that has been treated with a commercial lactase enzyme product to reduce the lactose content. Refer to the section on lactose intolerance for further information.

Sample High-Energy High-Protein Restricted-Lactose Full Fluid Diet (Strict)

Meal	Food Item	Amount	Energy kJ	Energy kcal	Protein (g)
Breakfast	Orange juice with	125 mL ($\frac{1}{2}$ cup)	230	55	1
	Polycose*	15 mL (1 tbsp)	125	30	0
	Treated[†] whole milk	250 mL (1 cup)	670	160	8
	Strained oatmeal with	125 mL ($\frac{1}{2}$ cup)	295	70	2
	Milk-free margarine	10 mL (2 tsp)	315	75	0
	and Brown sugar	15 mL (1 tbsp)	140	34	0
Snack	Vanilla Ensure Plus®*	250 mL (1 cup/ 1 can)	1490	355	13
Lunch	Apple juice with	125 mL ($\frac{1}{2}$ cup)	250	60	0.5
	Polycose*	15 mL (1 tbsp)	125	30	0
	Treated[†] whole milk	250 mL (1 cup)	670	160	8
	Tomato soup made with				
	Treated[†] milk and	250 mL (1 cup)	715	170	6
	Milk-free margarine	15 mL (1 tbsp)	420	100	0
	Orange gelatin	125 mL ($\frac{1}{2}$ cup)	315	75	2
Snack	Chocolate Ensure Plus®*	250 mL (1 cup/ 1 can)	1490	355	13
Evening meal	Tomato juice	125 mL ($\frac{1}{2}$ cup)	85	20	1
	Treated[†] whole milk	250 mL (1 cup)	670	160	8
	Strained beef soup with	250 mL (1 cup)	170	40	4
	Milk-free margarine	10 mL (2 tsp)	315	75	0
	Vanilla pudding made with treated[†] whole milk	125 mL ($\frac{1}{2}$ cup)	840	200	3
Snack	Strawberry Ensure Plus®*	250 mL (1 cup/ 1 can)	1490	355	13
Total			10820	2580	82.5

* Or equivalent. Refer to the section on commercial supplements.

† Treated milk refers to milk that has been treated with a commercial lactase enzyme product to reduce the lactose content. Refer to the dietary modifications section for further information on lactose intolerance.

- Strained cream and stock soups (mildly seasoned only)
- Strained, cooked refined cereals such as Cream of Wheat™, Cream of Rice™, oatmeal
- Most commercial supplements (refer to the section on commercial supplements)

TIPS TO IMPROVE THE NUTRITIONAL VALUE OF THE FULL FLUID DIET

- Use higher-fat dairy products such as whole milk and cream in place of 2 percent or skim milk.
- Use butter or margarine in cooked refined hot cereals and soups.
- Add skim milk powder to hot cereals, milk, cream soups, yogurt, puddings, and so forth.
- Incorporate commercial supplements into the daily diet (as required).
- Take a well-balanced multivitamin and mineral supplement daily.

LIGHT OR BLAND DIET

Individuals with IBD may be advised to follow a light or bland diet. In general, this is a diet consisting of foods that are easy to digest and devoid of foods considered to be gas forming. Foods allowed are mildly seasoned, and moderately low in fat and fiber. Rather than three meals per day, six smaller, more frequent meals are encouraged. This diet is based on traditional dietary practices rather than on scientific evidence of efficacy and does not take into consideration individual tolerances and intolerances. If it is followed for a long period, this diet has the potential to cause nutrient imbalance and deficiency, thus failing to meet the increased needs of individuals with active disease.

FOODS TO AVOID

- Spices such as black or red pepper
- Highly seasoned foods such as spiced meat, fish, poultry, soups, salad dressings, cheese
- Caffeine-containing foods such as coffee, strong tea, carbonated cola beverages, and chocolate
- Alcohol
- Fiber-containing foods such as fruits and vegetables with seeds, tough skins, or membranes
- Potentially gas-forming vegetables such as broccoli, brussels sprouts, cabbage, cauliflower, onions, radishes, turnips, dried beans and peas
- All breads, cereals, and baked products made from whole grains
- All nuts and seeds

Although there is no evidence that this diet is of special value to individuals with IBD, it may be more palatable and better tolerated than a regular diet during an acute attack of IBD. Foods to be avoided vary with each individual, so you should discuss the matter with your physician and registered dietitian, especially if you follow the diet on a regular or frequent basis.

RESTRICTED-LACTOSE DIET

Lactose, the natural sugar found in milk and milk products, is digested in the small intestine by an enzyme called *lactase*. Lactase splits lactose into the digestible sugars glucose and galactose, which are easily absorbed from the intestine. In some individuals, the body does not produce sufficient quantities of this enzyme, and when milk or milk products are consumed, the lactose remains in the intestinal tract undigested. This undigested lactose causes water to be drawn into the intestine. Undigested lactose also serves as an energy source for intestinal bacteria. As a result, an insufficiency of lactase produces symptoms of gas, gut rumblings, cramps, bloating, and diarrhea. The inability to digest and absorb lactose is called *lactose intolerance.*

Lactose intolerance can be primary or secondary. Primary lactose intolerance is a permanent loss of the enzyme lactase, which may be present at birth or arise in the early years. Most races have a significant incidence of primary lactose intolerance. Blacks, Asians, Orientals, and North and South American Natives have a higher incidence of lactose intolerance than do Caucasians. Secondary lactose intolerance may arise because of injury or other illness in the gastrointestinal tract. Possible causes include intestinal infections, active Crohn's disease involving the upper small intestine, or the use of medications such as antibiotics (substances that interfere with the growth of microorganisms). In secondary lactose intolerance, the inability to digest lactose is temporary. Although it was once thought that the incidence of lactose intolerance was greater in individuals with IBD, this is now known not to be true. IBD and lactose intolerance do not go hand in hand, but an individual may have both IBD and lactose intolerance.

Primary lactose intolerance can often be diagnosed simply from a history of symptoms following the ingestion of milk. Some individuals may have symptoms for many years. Secondary lactose intolerance, which may arise in active IBD, is more difficult to diagnose because the symptoms of lactose intolerance and active disease can overlap. In general, unless one has a primary lactose intolerance, one tolerates lactose well during periods of active IBD. Because milk and milk products are an important source of protein, calcium, and energy, it is essential that these foods not be excluded from the diet unnecessarily. If you are concerned that you might have lactose intolerance, you are encouraged to discuss this with your physician and registered dietitian. Specific tests are available to identify a lactose intolerance.

RESTRICTED-LACTOSE DIET—GENERAL GUIDELINES

If you have a documented primary or secondary lactose intolerance, the following information will be helpful to you. If the lactose intolerance is significant, you are encouraged to seek further advice from a registered dietitian.

- The tolerance to lactose varies among individuals. To establish your tolerance level, initially restrict all lactose-containing foods. Gradually add small amounts of lactose-containing foods to identify tolerance. For some individuals, only large intakes of lactose give rise to adverse symptoms, but for others, any amount of lactose results in distress.
- Commercial enzymatic products are available. These products hydrolyze the lactose in milk and milk products. Such products are available in a liquid form, to be used to treat milk; in a tablet form, to be taken before consuming lactose-containing foods; and as pre-treated milk.
- Lactose is found in milk and milk products. Avoid fluid milk, evaporated milk, powdered milk, buttermilk, goats' milk, cream, or any products to which milk has been added. This includes cream soup, ice milk, ice cream, pudding, and so forth, unless the milk has been treated with a commercial lactase enzyme product.
- Read product labels. Lactose may be added during the processing of a food or drug. Generally, avoid products containing lactose, milk, milk solids, skim milk powder, cream, evaporated milk, condensed milk, whey, and curds.
- Fermented products, such as yogurt, may be well tolerated. However, milk, cream, or milk solids are often added after the fermentation process to reduce the sour taste. This may result in a significant lactose content. Read the label.
- Unless you are highly lactose intolerant, you can probably safely eat natural cheeses that have been aged because the lactose content is minimal. Such cheeses include bleu, brick, Camembert, Cheddar, Colby, Edam, provolone, and Swiss.
- If you are highly lactose intolerant, you may need to avoid breads and baked products if they contain lactose. Read the label.
- Lactose-containing foods may be better tolerated if small amounts are taken throughout the day rather than as a large quantity at one time.
- Lactose is generally better tolerated if taken with a meal rather than alone as a beverage or a snack.
- Liquid soy milk is a lactose-free milk substitute that tastes good and can be used in many recipes in place of milk.
- Lactose-free commercial supplements can replace regular milk in most recipes. If you require a commercial supplement, choose one that is lactose free. Refer to the section on commercial supplements for further information.
- Further advice should be sought from a registered dietitian, especially if you have a significant lactose intolerance.

Sample Restricted-Lactose Diet (Strict)

Meal	Food Item	Amount
Breakfast	Orange juice	125 mL ($\frac{1}{2}$ cup)
	Treated* milk	250 mL (1 cup)
	Enriched whole-grain	
	bread (milk-free) with	2 slices
	Milk-free margarine	15 mL (1 tbsp)
	Poached egg	1
Lunch	Tossed green salad with lemon	180 mL ($\frac{3}{4}$ cup)
	Cheese sandwich:	
	Cheddar cheese	30 g (1 oz)
	Whole-wheat bread (milk-free)	2 slices
	Milk-free margarine	5–10 mL (1–2 tsp)
	Apple	1 medium
Snack	Dinner roll (milk-free) with	1
	Milk-free margarine	5–10 mL (1–2 tsp)
Evening meal	Treated* milk	250 mL (1 cup)
	Roast beef	90 g (3 oz)
	Baked potato with	1 medium
	Milk-free margarine	5–10 mL (1–2 tsp)
	Boiled carrots	125 mL ($\frac{1}{2}$ cup)
	Vanilla pudding made with	
	treated* milk	125 mL ($\frac{1}{2}$ cup)

* Treated milk refers to milk that has been treated with a commercial lactase enzyme product to reduce the lactose content.

RESTRICTED-FAT DIET

A restricted-fat diet is usually unnecessary for IBD patients. This is especially true if you are underweight, since a restricted-fat diet may severely limit energy intake and contribute to further weight loss. However, if your weight is within the recommended range and your disease is not active, a lower-fat diet is a good way to reduce energy intake and promote a healthy weight and lifestyle. In Crohn's disease, a restricted-fat diet may be necessary if fat malabsorption has been diagnosed by your physician. The following are general guidelines for a fat-restricted diet if required on a temporary or permanent basis. You are encouraged to seek further advice from your physician and registered dietitian if the restriction is to be prolonged.

RESTRICTED-FAT DIET—GENERAL GUIDELINES

- Avoid all fried foods.
- If you must fry, use a non-stick frying pan. Do not add fat, and drain off fat from frying meat as it collects in the pan.
- To remove excess fat from soups, stews and other dishes, prepare them a day ahead, refrigerate, and remove hardened fat that has collected on the surface.
- Choose lean meats, trimming away all visible fat.
- Use cooking methods that remove fat, such as boiling, broiling, barbecuing, or baking.
- Limit the use of visible fat, such as butter, margarine, gravy, lard, vegetable oil, salad dressings, visible fat on meat, and skin on chicken.
- Avoid regular luncheon meat, unless the package indicates low fat content.
- Read labels and limit any commercial products such as pastries and baking mixes that contain significant amounts of butter, margarine, shortening, oil, or lard. Ingredients are listed in order of amount. The further down on the list an ingredient appears, the smaller the amount of the ingredient in the product. Therefore, look for products where fat is near the end of the list.
- Choose lower-fat dairy products. When reading a label, choose a product that is lowest in butter fat (B.F.) or milk fat (M.F.). For example, choose skim, 1 percent or 2 percent milk, yogurt, and cottage cheese. When buying a cheese, choose one that contains less than 20 percent M.F. or B.F.
- In many recipes, ingredients such as butter, margarine, and oil can be reduced by 25 percent or more. Experiment with your favorite recipes to obtain an acceptable lower-fat product.

Low-Fat High-Energy Suggestions

Food Item	Use In/On
Sugar, honey	Fruit, fruit juices, tea and coffee, hot and cold cereals, glaze for meats such as ham and chicken, sweet sauces for meats and fruits
Jam, jelly, syrup	Sherbet, low-fat yogurt, breads, toast, hot and cold cereals, glaze for meats such as ham, sweet sauces for meats and fruits
Dried fruit	Low-fat muffins and sweet breads, hot and cold cereals, sweet sauces for meats or desserts, puddings made with skim milk, rice dishes

Low-Fat High-Protein Suggestions

Food Item	Use In/On
Skim milk powder	Fluid milk, soups, low-fat sauces and creamed entrées or vegetables, low-fat puddings and custards, low-fat dips
Skim milk	Cooked cereals (use for cooking instead of water), soups, low-fat sauces and creamed entrées or vegetables, low-fat puddings and custards
Low-fat cottage cheese	Jellied salads, fruit, baked potatoes, low-fat dips, low-fat pancakes and casseroles
Low-fat yogurt	Cooked cereal, fruit, flavored gelatin, as a substitute for sour cream in recipes and dips
Instant breakfast	Skim milk
Low-fat cheese	Toast, sandwiches, salads, grated on vegetables, casseroles, stews, and soups

Low-Fat Snack Suggestions

Milk Group
Puddings made with skim milk
Low-fat yogurt, plain or with fruit
Low-fat cottage cheese, plain or with fruit

Bread/Cereal Group
Plain angel food cake
Toast, soda crackers, melba toast with jam
 or honey
Cold cereal and skim milk alone or topped
 with fruit
Arrowroot cookies
Bread sticks
Graham crackers

Meat/Alternate Group
Low-fat cheese plain or on soda crackers
Low-fat cheese melted on bread or bagels

Fruit/Vegetable Group
Fruit juice
Fruit juice popsicles
Jellied fruit salad
Dried fruit mixed with plain yogurt
Fresh fruit
Canned fruit served over sherbet
Fresh vegetables with a yogurt dip

Extra
Marshmallows, hard or jellied candies, sherbet, fruit ices, flavored gelatin

Sample Restricted-Fat Diet

Meal	Food Item	Amount	Energy kJ	kcal	Fat (g)
Breakfast	Orange juice	125 mL ($\frac{1}{2}$ cup)	230	55	0
	Skim milk	250 mL (1 cup)	380	90	0
	Whole-wheat bread with	2 slices	525	125	2
	Butter	5 mL (1 tsp)	150	36	4
	Poached egg	1	335	80	6
	Tea	250 mL (1 cup)	0	0	0
Lunch	Tossed green salad with	180 mL ($\frac{3}{4}$ cup)	42	10	0
	Vinegar	2 mL ($\frac{1}{2}$ tsp)	0	0	0
	Cheese sandwich:				
	Part-skim mozzarella	30 g (1 oz)	335	80	4.7
	Whole-wheat bread	2 slices	525	125	2
	Butter	5 mL (1 tsp)	150	36	4
	Apple	1 medium	335	80	0
Snack	Whole-grain roll with	1	650	155	2
	Jam	15 mL (1 tbsp)	230	55	0
Evening meal	Skim milk	250 mL (1 cup)	335	80	0
	Roast beef (lean)	90 g (3 oz)	735	175	7
	Baked potato with	1 medium	505	120	0
	Butter	5 mL (1 tsp)	150	36	4
	Boiled carrots with	125 mL ($\frac{1}{2}$ cup)	145	35	0
	Dill and lemon sprinkle		0	0	0
	Sherbet	125 mL ($\frac{1}{2}$ cup)	590	140	2
Total			6350	1515	38

FIBER-MODIFIED DIETS

Dietary fiber is the portion of a plant that the human body cannot digest. It provides undigestible bulk, which encourages the normal elimination of body wastes. It is not a single entity, but rather a mixture of several fibers that can be classified into two groups based on their solubility in water. *Soluble fiber* includes pectin, gums, and mucilage. These readily dissolve in water to form a gel that slows gastric emptying and binds bile acids but has little effect on stool size. Soluble fiber is found in significant quantities in beans, oats, and some fruits and vegetables.

Insoluble fiber includes cellulose, hemicellulose, and lignin. These fibers do not dissolve in water, but they do possess considerable water-retaining capacity. This water-retaining property, referred to as the *bulking effect,* provides for softer, bulkier stools that pass through the bowel faster and are excreted without straining. Insoluble fiber is found in fruit and vegetable pulp and their skins, stalks, and leaves and in the outer coatings of grains, nuts, seeds, and legumes. Meat and other animal products do not contain fiber. Cooking or blenderizing food does not reduce the total fiber content but may affect how quickly and easily the food is digested.

It is estimated that the diet of the average North American contains 15 to 20 g of fiber per day. The actual amount of fiber that should be included in the diet on a daily basis is unknown. Research has indicated that diets low in fiber are linked to cancer of the colon, diverticular disease (herniations, or outpouchings, of the wall

Fiber Content of Some Common Foods

Food Group	Food Item	Serving Size	Fiber (g)
Milk group	All	Any amount	0
Meat/alternate group	Meat, fish, poultry	Any amount	0
	Baked beans	250 mL (1 cup)	14.6
	Lentils, cooked	250 mL (1 cup)	7.8
	Peanut butter	60 mL ($\frac{1}{4}$ cup)	4.8
Bread/cereal group	Bran buds	175 mL ($\frac{3}{4}$ cup)	14.9
	Bran flakes	175 mL ($\frac{3}{4}$ cup)	3.7
	Corn flakes	175 mL ($\frac{3}{4}$ cup)	0.1
	Wheat, puffed	250 mL (1 cup)	0.6
	Bran muffin	1 average	2.5
	Bread, whole-wheat	1 slice	1.4
	Bread, white	1 slice	0.4
	Macaroni, cooked	125 mL ($\frac{1}{2}$ cup)	0.3
Fruit/vegetable group	Prunes, stewed	125 mL ($\frac{1}{2}$ cup)	8.3
	Apple	1 medium	3.5
	Orange	1 medium	2.6
	Banana	$\frac{1}{2}$ large	1.2
	Peas, cooked	125 mL ($\frac{1}{2}$ cup)	3.8
	Potato, mashed	125 mL ($\frac{1}{2}$ cup)	1.1
	Corn, cooked	125 mL ($\frac{1}{2}$ cup)	2.4
	Spinach, cooked	125 mL ($\frac{1}{2}$ cup)	2.3
	Carrot, cooked	1 medium	2.2
	Lettuce, shredded	125 mL ($\frac{1}{2}$ cup)	0.5

of the gastrointestinal tract), constipation (irregular, difficult, or sluggish passage of stool), and heart disease. Because of the possible associations with these ailments, general dietary guidelines for healthy individuals suggests a doubling of the present intake, or a daily consumption of 30 to 40 g of fiber each day. As noted below, this amount of dietary fiber may be unwise in some individuals with IBD. All types of fiber are important, so both soluble and insoluble fiber from all food sources is encouraged. Following the food guides, which encourage the consumption of fruits, vegetables, and whole grains, will help you achieve a healthy intake of fiber.

RESTRICTED-FIBER DIET

Over time, the knowledge of the role of fiber in IBD and health care based thereupon have undergone change. In the past, a restricted-fiber diet was thought to be necessary for all individuals with IBD, and such diets were regularly prescribed as a standard part of medical care. Restricting the amount of fiber in the diet and reducing the amount of stool produced was considered to be beneficial for the damaged bowel. Some health care workers believed that such a regimen would also control the disease activity. However, evidence has shown that reducing dietary fiber has no effect on preventing relapses (the reinitiation of active disease

---

RESTRICTED-FIBER DIET—GENERAL GUIDELINES

- Follow the food guides to ensure that you are meeting your nutrient needs.
- All milk and milk products such as ice cream, yogurt, and cheese are allowed. Avoid any product that contains seeds, nuts, or skins.
- All meat, fish, poultry, and eggs are allowed.
- Avoid meat alternatives, such as cooked dried beans, peas, lentils, nuts, or seeds.
- Choose breads and cereals made from refined white flour and cereals. Avoid products made from whole-grain flours or cereals and those containing nuts, seeds, or skins.
- Limit fruit and vegetable intake to two servings of each per day. Refer to the food guide for serving sizes.
- Avoid all dried fruits.
- Remove the skin and seeds of fruits and vegetables.
- Avoid prune juice. All other juices are allowed and encouraged as an excellent low-fiber source of nutrients.
- Avoid higher-fiber vegetables such as broccoli, spinach, corn, peas, and brussels sprouts.

after a period of inactive disease). In fact, such a fiber-restricted regimen could be detrimental. A fiber-restricted diet can be nutritionally inadequate because dietary intake of vitamin C, folic acid, zinc, and other nutrients may be below optimal levels. Since good nutrition is essential to good health, more recent recommendations encourage the consumption of a well-balanced diet, including fiber-rich foods, as indicated in the food guides and as tolerated. This should be the primary focus of dietary manipulation. Unless specifically advised by your physician and registered dietitian, you should not consume a fiber-restricted diet. If you are presently following a self-prescribed fiber-restricted diet and are considering modifying your diet to include more fiber, you should discuss your diet with your doctor and registered dietitian before making any changes.

As much as an unrestricted, well-balanced diet is encouraged, certain situations may require some degree of short-term fiber restriction. Acute active disease

Sample Restricted-Fiber Diet

Meal	Food Item	Amount	Fiber (g)
Breakfast	Orange juice	125 mL ($\frac{1}{2}$ cup)	0
	2% milk	250 mL (1 cup)	0
	Enriched white bread with	2 slices	0.8
	Butter	5–10 mL (1–2 tsp)	0
	Poached egg	1	0
Snack	Apple juice	125 mL ($\frac{1}{2}$ cup)	0
Lunch	Tomato juice	125 mL ($\frac{1}{2}$ cup)	0
	Cheese sandwich:		
	Cheese	30 g (1 oz)	0
	Enriched white bread	2 slices	0.8
	Butter	5–10 mL (1–2 tsp)	0
	Peeled apple	1 medium	2
Snack	Enriched white roll with	1	1
	Margarine	5–10 mL (1–2 tsp)	0
Evening meal	2% milk	250 mL (1 cup)	0
	Roast beef	90 g (3 oz)	0
	Boiled peeled potato with	1 medium	1.4
	Butter	5–10 mL (1–2 tsp)	0
	Boiled Carrots	125 mL ($\frac{1}{2}$ cup)	2.5
	Sherbet	125 mL ($\frac{1}{2}$ cup)	0
Total			8.5

of the colon is often associated with diarrhea, abdominal cramps, pain, and rectal bleeding. To some extent, a restricted-fiber diet may help to reduce some of these symptoms. Once these symptoms have improved, a normal fiber intake should be gradually resumed to promote optimal nutritional intake. As noted previously, there is no evidence that fiber restriction should be continued in chronic disease, especially if the individual is free of symptoms. Acute active Crohn's disease of the small bowel may also necessitate some degree of fiber restriction. The inflammatory process associated with acute disease may result in significant intestinal narrowing, which can contribute to cramping, pain, and diarrhea after eating. Once the in-flammatory process subsides, a slow increase in dietary fiber to a normal intake is suggested. In Crohn's disease, if chronic inflammation has resulted in stricture formation (the abnormal narrowing of a passage caused by scar tissue) in the small or large bowel, the avoidance of high-fiber foods on a long-term basis may be necessary to prevent blockage and to reduce cramping. If you have been advised to follow a restricted-fiber diet, it is important to make wise food choices to ensure that your nutrient needs are being met. If you cannot follow a well-balanced diet as outlined in the food guide, a well-balanced multivitamin and mineral supplement is advisable. Often, the advice of a registered dietitian is helpful.

HIGH-FIBER DIET

Although much attention centers on the management of diarrhea, some individuals with IBD suffer from constipation. The definition of constipation is varied, but the condition can be generally described as the irregular, difficult, or sluggish passage of stools. Often stools are dry, small in size, and difficult to expel. Constipation can be an infrequent problem or an ongoing daily concern and can be caused by a number of disorders. Constipation can be the side effect of medications that affect the rate of intestinal transit; it can result from a disorder of bowel structure such as a stricture; or it may be the result of an improper diet. Constipation can also be a learned behavior. For example, some individuals with hemorrhoids or anal fissures (an ulcer, crack, or break in the wall of the anus) choose to ignore the "urge to go" and retain stool rather than experience the pain associated with passing stool. The end result of this practice is a worsening of the constipation and more discomfort on defecation (evacuation of the bowels). A frequent contributor to the development of constipation is a lack of fiber in the diet. Insoluble fiber absorbs water, which increases the bulk of the stool and provides the stimulus for normal contractions and movement in the colon. Without this stimulus, stool passes very slowly along the gastrointestinal tract, allowing more opportunity for water reabsorption, resulting in the development of small, dry stools that may be difficult to pass.

In IBD, the treatment for constipation involves medical investigation to rule out an underlying physical cause. In many cases, the constipation is simply caused by inadequate dietary habits, and a high-fiber diet is prescribed as the treatment. The exact amount of fiber that is required to alleviate constipation is varied. Some individuals require about 25 g per day to have regular bowel movements, whereas others require double this amount. Of the various fibers, wheat bran, which is composed mainly of cellulose, is one of the more effective stool-softening fibers. However, a wide variety of fiber from different food sources should be consumed. To ensure adequate fluid to allow for stool bulking, six to eight glasses of water should be included in the diet every day. When a high-fiber diet is initiated, it is important to slowly increase the fiber intake to allow the gastrointestinal tract to adjust. A sudden increase in dietary fiber can cause gas, abdominal discomfort, and possibly diarrhea. As with many other nutrients, it is possible to consume too much fiber. An excessive fiber intake is thought to interfere with the absorption of iron, calcium, and other nutrients.

In addition to increasing the fiber content of the diet, other lifestyle modifications are needed for the prevention of constipation. It is important to develop

GENERAL GUIDELINES AND TIPS FOR INCREASING DIETARY FIBER INTAKE

- Milk and milk products, meat, fish, poultry, cheese, and eggs do not contain fiber but are a part of a balanced diet.
- Meat alternates such as nuts, seeds, peanut butter, cooked dried peas, beans, and lentils are an excellent source of fiber. Add nuts and seeds to salads, muffins, rice, and casseroles; add chick peas or kidney beans to salads or casseroles.
- Whole-grain food choices from the bread/cereal group are an excellent source of fiber. Choose 100 percent whole-wheat bread, bran muffins, whole-wheat pasta, and bran cereals; sprinkle raw bran or a bran cereal in soups, hot cereals, baked products, and meat loaf.
- Choose fresh raw fruit and vegetables in place of juice.
- Add dried fruit to yogurt, hot and cold cereals, rice, and muffins.
- Choose baked products that utilize fruits and vegetables such as zucchini loaf, carrot cake, and so on.
- Increase the fiber content of the diet slowly to help reduce potential adverse effects such as abdominal bloating and gas.
- Distribute high-fiber foods evenly throughout the day.
- Drink six to eight glasses of fluid daily.
- Avoid any high-fiber food that consistently gives rise to adverse affects.

regular bowel and health habits. This includes learning to respond to the signals for defecation and to pass stools when the urge is present. Eating balanced meals, as outlined in the food guides, on a regular basis and taking the time to incorporate exercise into your daily schedule is also important. Such modifications may take months to achieve but are necessary changes for individuals with frequent constipation.

If you suffer from constipation or are interested in following a higher-fiber diet, you are advised to consult your physician and registered dietitian before making any extensive dietary changes. It is essential to ensure that the constipation is not related to a more serious medical concern and that a higher-fiber diet will not be problematic.

Sample High-Fiber Diet

Meal	Food Item	Amount	Fiber (g)
Breakfast	Orange	1 medium	2.6
	2% milk	250 mL (1 cup)	0
	Whole-wheat bread with	1 slice	1.4
	Butter	5 mL (1 tsp)	0
	All-bran cereal	125 mL ($\frac{1}{2}$ cup)	9.9
	Poached egg	1 medium	0
Lunch	Tossed salad with	250 mL (1 cup)	1.4
	Mayonnaise and	15 mL (1 tbsp)	0
	Sesame seeds	15 mL (1 tbsp)	1
	Cheese sandwich:		
	Cheese	30 g (1 oz)	0
	Whole-wheat bread	2 slices	2.8
	Butter	5–10 mL (1–2 tsp)	0
	Apple	1 medium	3.2
Snack	Bran muffin with	1 medium	3.5
	Peanut butter	30 mL (2 tbsp)	2.1
Evening meal	Sliced tomato	$\frac{1}{2}$ medium	1.5
	2% milk	250 mL (1 cup)	0
	Roast beef	90 g (3 oz)	0
	Baked potato (with skin) with	1 medium	3
	Butter	5–10 mL (1–2 tsp)	0
	Cooked peas	125 mL ($\frac{1}{2}$ cup)	4.6
	Sherbet	125 mL ($\frac{1}{2}$ cup)	0
Total			37

HIGH-CALCIUM DIET

Calcium needs are increased in individuals who are taking corticosteroid medications such as prednisone. These drugs decrease the intestinal absorption of calcium and increase the risk of development of osteoporosis. If you are taking prednisone on a regular basis, ensure a good intake of calcium-rich foods daily. Aim for a daily intake of 1200 to 1500 mg of calcium.

Calcium Content of Selected Foods

Food Group	Food Item	Amount	Calcium (mg)
Milk group	Milk, 2%	250 mL (1 cup)	315
	Milk, skim, powder	80 mL ($\frac{1}{3}$ cup)	308
	Yogurt, plain	125 mL ($\frac{1}{2}$ cup)	215
	Cheese, cheddar	45 g ($1\frac{1}{2}$ oz)	324
Meat/alternate group	Sardines, canned, with bones	7 medium	367
	Salmon, canned, with bones	90 g (3 oz)	146
	Almonds	125 mL ($\frac{1}{2}$ cup)	200
	Tofu	90 g (3 oz)	100
Fruit/vegetable group	Broccoli, raw	1 medium stalk	72
	Spinach, cooked	125 mL ($\frac{1}{2}$ cup)	126
Bread/cereal group	Bread, white, calcium carbonate added	1 slice	46
Extra	Molasses, blackstrap	15 mL (1 tbsp)	144

SUGGESTIONS FOR IMPROVING CALCIUM INTAKE

- When making cream soup, dilute canned condensed soup with milk, instead of water.
- Add skim milk powder to hot cereal, sauces, soups, casseroles, milk, baked products.
- Add grated cheese to salads, soups, casseroles, vegetables.
- Add a slice of cheese to sandwiches, hamburgers, or apple pie.

(Continued)

(Continued)
- Choose yogurt, milk puddings, cheese and crackers, milk, or milkshakes as a snack.
- In recipes for vegetable dip, use yogurt in place of sour cream.
- Use a milk or cheese sauce for broccoli, brussels sprouts, cauliflower.
- Grilled cheese sandwiches or toasted bagels with melted cheese make an excellent high-calcium breakfast, lunch, or snack.
- Do not remove the bones from canned salmon because they are an excellent source of calcium. Crush and mix the bones into the salmon meat. Use for salmon sandwiches, salmon loaf, or salmon salad.

IRON-RICH DIET

Iron deficiency affects a large portion of the general population in addition to individuals with IBD. Women are particularly at risk because of the regular blood loss that occurs during menstruation. Men and women with IBD can become iron deficient because of chronic blood loss from the gastrointestinal tract in conjunction with a poor dietary iron intake. In order to ensure good stores of this important nutrient, you should incorporate iron-rich foods into your diet on a regular basis.

TIPS TO IMPROVE IRON INTAKE

- Follow the food guides to help plan well-balanced, nutritious meals.
- Choose both animal- and plant-source iron-rich foods as often as possible.
- Include an iron-rich animal-source food at every meal.
- Include a source of vitamin C such as orange juice at every meal to enhance iron absorption.
- Avoid drinking coffee or tea with meals as this reduces the absorption of iron.
- Incorporate iron-rich foods into cooking and baking to enhance the iron content:
  - Add dried fruit to muffins, quick breads, hot and cold cereals.
  - Add chick peas to casseroles and salads, or blenderize and use as a vegetable dip.
  - Add extra kidney beans to chili, stews, dried bean salads.
  - When muffin and quick bread recipes call for dry cereal, add iron-enriched cereals.
  - Spinach can be chopped and added to soups, salads, and stir-fried vegetable dishes.
  - Add clams to seafood casserole dishes.
- Use iron pots and pans to cook foods.

Sources of Dietary Iron

Food Item	Amount	Iron (mg)
Pork/calves liver, cooked	90 g (3 oz)	13–15
Pumpkin seeds, dried	125 mL ($\frac{1}{2}$ cup)	10
Beef heart/kidney, cooked	90 g (3 oz)	6.5–7
Oysters, raw	90 g (3 oz)	5
Chick peas, cooked	250 mL (1 cup)	5.2
Red kidney beans, cooked	250 mL (1 cup)	4.7
Lima beans, cooked	250 mL (1 cup)	4.4
Blackstrap molasses	15 mL (1 tbsp)	3.4
Clams, canned	90 g (3 oz)	3.3
Lean beef/veal, cooked	90 g (3 oz)	3.0
Enriched cold cereals	250 mL (1 cup)	3–8
Enriched pasta, cooked	250 mL (1 cup)	2.5
Dried fruit (raisins, apricots, etc.)	125 mL ($\frac{1}{2}$ cup)	2–5
Spinach, cooked	125 mL ($\frac{1}{2}$ cup)	2
Bran muffin	1 medium	1.3
Egg, whole	1 large	1.2
Whole-wheat/enriched white bread	1 slice	0.6

HIGH-ENERGY DIET

The most common nutritional problem in individuals with IBD is an inadequate energy intake, which leads to weight loss and muscle wasting. Pain, diarrhea, and a general disinterest in food are all major contributing factors. Weight loss, especially during active disease, interferes with the body's ability to function efficiently and hinders the capability to fight infection and to heal. Weight loss resulting in a chronic state of underweight (less than 90 percent of ideal weight for height, age, and body build) interferes with the ability to regain good health during even minor illnesses such as the common cold or flu. In addition, being chronically underweight affects general energy levels, strength, and positive body self-image.

Although many individuals with IBD feel that being underweight is an inevitable consequence of the disease process, this is not true. In IBD, being underweight is often a contributing factor in a vicious circle. During active disease, a lack of energy and a general poor sense of well-being leads to a reduced nutrient intake, resulting in weight loss and a loss of muscle. This loss of weight and muscle further contributes to tiredness and a lack of motivation, which inevitably leads to a further reduction in nutrient intake. Once this cycle is started, it is difficult to halt, and it eventually leads to underweight and general poor health. The best way to address this problem is to prevent the process from starting. It is much easier to maintain a good weight than to correct for losses. Prevention is the key. Preventing weight loss or achieving weight gain requires knowledge and motivation. Often only a few minor adjustments in daily eating habits will result in achieving a healthy weight.

How much you should weigh and how much you need to eat to achieve a good weight are unique to every individual. Your ideal body weight (the recom-

---

CALCULATING IDEAL BODY WEIGHT FOR WOMEN

Step 1

- For 5 feet of height, allow 100 pounds.
- For each additional inch of height, add 5 pounds.
- For each inch of height under 5 feet, subtract 5 pounds.

EXAMPLE: If you are 5 feet 3 inches,

• First 5 feet	100 pounds
• Additional 3 inches	+15 pounds
• Ideal body weight	115 pounds

Step 2

- If you have a large body frame, add 10 percent of your calculated weight.
- If you have a small frame, subtract 10 percent of you calculated weight.
- If you are an average frame your ideal weight is as calculated.

EXAMPLE: If you have a small frame,

• Calculated ideal body weight	115 pounds
• Subtract 10 percent of calculated ideal weight	−11 pounds
• Ideal body weight for small frame	104 pounds

EXAMPLE: If you have a large frame,

• Calculated ideal body weight	115 pounds
• Add 10 percent of calculated ideal weight	+11 pounds
• Ideal body weight for large frame	126 pounds

Note: To convert to kilograms (kg), divide your weight in pounds by 2.2.

mended weight for height and age that is associated with good health) depends on a number of factors such as the size of your frame or your bone structure, age, and body composition (percentage of muscle versus fat). Bone weighs more than muscle, which weighs more than fat, so the larger your frame and the more muscular you are, the more you should weigh at any given height. Energy needs vary with gender, weight, age, body temperature, and physical activity. The more you weigh and the more the muscular you are, the more energy you require to maintain that weight and muscle tone. Because men tend to weigh more than women and have a greater percentage of muscle than women, men require more energy than

---

CALCULATING IDEAL BODY WEIGHT FOR MEN

Step 1

- For 5 feet of height, allow 105 pounds.
- For each additional inch of height, add 6 pounds.
- For each inch under 5 feet of height, subtract 6 pounds.

EXAMPLE: If you are 5 feet 10 inches,

• First 5 feet	105 pounds
• Additional 10 inches	+60 pounds
• Ideal body weight	165 pounds

Step 2

- If you have a large body frame, add 10 percent to your calculated ideal weight.
- If you have a small frame, subtract 10 percent of your calculated ideal weight.
- If you have an average frame your weight is as calculated.

EXAMPLE: If you have a small frame,

• Calculated ideal body weight	165 pounds
• Subtract 10 percent of calculated weight	−16 pounds
• Ideal body weight for small frame	149 pounds

EXAMPLE: If you have a large frame,

• Calculated ideal body weight	165 pounds
• Add 10 percent of calculated weight	+16 pounds
• Ideal body weight for large frame	181 pounds

Note: To convert to kilograms (kg), divide your weight in pounds by 2.2.

Calculating Energy Needs

| Activity Level | Example | Activity Factor | |
		Males	Females
Sedentary	Office worker Student	16	13
Moderately active	Waitress in busy café Regular exercise routine	20	16
Very active	Professional athlete Construction worker	25	21

women. Changes in body composition and activity associated with aging results in decreased energy needs. Body temperature also affects energy needs. For individuals with IBD, energy needs increase in association with a fever. Elevated temperatures for lengthy periods can significantly increase energy needs. If the increased needs are not accommodated through an increase in energy intake, weight loss will result. For most individuals, the greatest determinant of energy needs is physical activity. The more physically demanding the activity and the longer the activity is carried out, the greater the energy required.

Various methods including tables, calculations, and sophisticated measuring techniques are available to help determine ideal body weight and energy requirements. A registered dietitian is most helpful in identifying your ideal body weight, establishing a goal weight (a more realistic individualized weight), and providing practical advice to help you achieve and maintain a good weight. If you feel that you are underweight, you are encouraged to discuss your concerns with your physician and registered dietitian. The information in the boxes on pages 70 and 71 will help you determine if you are underweight, while the table above, in combination with the examples below, will provide you with a quick method to estimate your energy needs for maintenance and weight gain. This information is not intended to replace professional advice, but has been included to encourage you to take an interest in achieving a good weight.

Example: A 103 pound female office worker not involved in a regular exercise routine.

Activity Factor × Weight (pounds) = Daily energy requirement
   13   103   1340 kcal (5600 kJ)

Example: A 135 pound sedentary male student.

Activity Factor × Weight (pounds) = Daily energy requirement
16   135   2160 kcal (9000 kJ)

Example: A 140 pound female professional athlete.

Activity Factor × Weight (pounds) = Daily energy requirement
21   140   2940 kcal (12300 kJ)

The above calculation allows you to determine the amount of energy required to maintain your present weight. It is calculated in kilocalories (kcal) and converted to kilojoules (kJ) by multiplying kilocalories by 4.2. If your goal is to gain weight, you need to increase your daily energy intake above the maintenance level. A

High-Energy Suggestions

Food Item	Use In/On
Butter or margarine	Toast, bread, pancakes, muffins, hot cereal, soup, vegetables, rice, potatoes, entrées
Sour cream	Potatoes, raw and cooked vegetables, soup, meat, salads, sauces, dips, pierogies
Mayonnaise	Salads, deviled eggs, sandwich fillings, dips
Cream (half & half)	Soup, pudding, cereals, coffee, tea, hot chocolate
Whipping cream	Puddings, pie, fruit, gelatin, ice cream, and other desserts
Cream cheese	Bagels, muffins, raw fruits, raw vegetables
Ice cream	Milk shakes, fruit gelatin, pie, cake
Vegetable oil	Salad dressings, sautéed meat or vegetables
Dried fruits	Muffins, cookies, breads, cakes, cereals, puddings, ice cream
Sugar and honey	Cereals, milk drinks, fruit desserts, glaze for meats such as chicken or ham, tea, coffee
Gravy	Meats, potatoes, french fries, pierogies

TIPS TO AID WEIGHT GAIN

- Consume three meals and three snacks daily.
- At meals and snacks, always choose high-energy, high-protein foods.
- At meals and snacks, avoid low-energy, filling liquids such as tea, coffee, clear soups, and water. In their place, choose higher-energy fluids, such as whole milk, milk shakes, chocolate milk, or juice.
- Eat frequently, approximately every two hours, even if you are not hungry.
- On days when your appetite is strong, eat well.
- Choose your favorite foods frequently. Have these food readily available at all times.
- Make food preparation easy on days when your appetite is poor. Take advantage of time-saving appliances such as blenders, food processors, and microwaves.
- Choose convenience foods, and ready-to-eat foods such as canned puddings, T.V. dinners, and canned stews to reduce the "burden" of meal preparation.
- Be creative. Do not limit yourself to traditional meals or food. For example, have pizza at breakfast, pancakes at supper, and so on.
- If you feel full quickly, limit large amounts of bulky foods such as raw fruits and vegetables, and obtain their nutrients by drinking fruit and vegetable juices. Save juice for the end of the meal so that you do not fill up on liquid rather than solids.
- If your disease is active and you are not able to tolerate solids, temporarily reduce your diet to full fluids. Use the guidelines provided in the full fluids section to ensure a nutrient-rich intake that provides for adequate energy and protein.
- If your appetite is poor, as may occur in active disease, the following suggestions may be helpful.
    - Add seasonings such as lemon juice, mint, or basil to food to improve its taste and aroma.
    - Serve food in a pleasant, relaxed atmosphere. Play your favorite music in the background.
    - Vary the color and texture of foods served on a plate, and add garnishes to make the meal more appetizing.
    - Eat in your favorite restaurant, or order in your favorite meal.
    - Use odors to stimulate the appetite: home-baked bread, cakes, simmering stews, soups, and roasts. If food odors diminish your appetite, plan cold items such as cottage cheese with fruit, cheese, cold meats, and salads for meals.
    - Invite a friend over to share meal time.
- Monitor your weight on a regular basis. If you start to lose weight, immediately alter your diet to increase your energy intake. The guidelines noted above will be helpful. If your weight continues to decrease, arrange to see your physician and registered dietitian to discuss the problem.

reasonable goal is to aim for a weight gain of $\frac{1}{2}$ to 1 kg (1 to 2 pounds) per week. To achieve this, you must consume an extra 2100 to 4200 kJ (500 to 1000 kcal) each day.

Example: A 103-pound female office worker leading a sedentary lifestyle. Goal is to gain weight.

Daily energy needs to maintain weight	5600 kJ (1340 kcal)
Daily energy needs to gain 1/2 kg (1 pound) per week	+2100 kJ (500 kcal)
	7700 kJ (1840 kcal)

Example: A 135-pound sedentary male student. Goal is to gain weight.

Daily energy needs to maintain weight	9000 kJ (2160 kcal)
Daily energy needs to gain 1/2 kg (1 poUnd) per week	+2100 kJ (500 kcal)
	11100 kJ (2660 kcal)

Example: A 140-pound female professional athlete. Goal is to gain weight.

Daily energy needs to maintain weight	12300 kJ (2940 kcal)
Daily energy needs to gain 1/2 kg (1 pound) per week	+2100 kJ (500 kcal)
	14400 kJ (3440 kcal)

Attempting to consume the amount of energy necessary for weight gain can sometimes seem overwhelming. The key to a successful weight gain program is to always choose high-energy foods and to persevere in increasing energy intake. Foods that are higher in fat are higher in energy at the same volume. For example, a glass of whole milk has twice the energy value as a glass of skim milk. The tips and suggestions on page 74 have been included to provide additional guidance. Sample high-energy, high-protein menus are found on pages 76–80 after the section entitled "High-Protein Diet." Note how subtle menu changes affect the total energy and protein levels.

HIGH-PROTEIN DIET

Protein deficiency is quite common in individuals with IBD. IN many situations it occurs concurrently with a need to increase energy intake, and, consequently, a high-energy diet and high-protein diet are often prescribed together. The following information offers general suggestions to aid in improving protein intake; protein is discussed in more detail in the section entitled "Macronutrients."

HIGH-PROTEIN DIET—GENERAL GUIDELINES

It is often helpful to incorporate protein-rich foods into other foods in order to concentrate nutritional value. This is especially valuable when appetite is poor and serving sizes are kept small.

Food Item	Suggestion
Milk	Use in milk shakes, creamed entrées, creamed vegetables, puddings, soups, sauces, custards.
Skim milk powder	Add to milk, cooked cereals, soups, puddings, casseroles, baked products such as muffins.
Eggs	Add finely chopped and blended into sauces and gravy. Add extra eggs in pancakes, muffins. Dip bread in eggs for french toast.
Cheese	Use in cream sauces for vegetables. Add grated or chopped to salad, omelets, potatoes, soups, noodle dishes, and so forth.
Cottage cheese	Use to make dips for fruit and vegetables. Add to pancake mix.
Meat, fish, poultry	Add cooked to soups, salads, casseroles, omelets, and so on.

High-Energy High-Protein Snack Ideas

Milk Group
Milk shake
Fruit yogurt
Milk pudding
Whole milk with added skim milk
Yogurt shake

Meat/Alternate Group
Cheese and crackers
Hard-cooked egg
Nuts
Peanut butter and crackers
4% cottage cheese topped with fruit
Egg salad, tuna salad, chicken salad sandwiches

Bread/Cereal Group
Toasted bagel with cheese
Muffin and cheese
Toasted English muffin with peanut butter
Corn chips topped with grated, melted cheese
Granola cereal with whole milk

Fruit/Vegetable Group
Assorted cheese and fruit tray
Celery sticks stuffed with peanut butter
Dried fruit added to fruit yogurt
Fresh fruit mixed with cottage cheese

Sample High-Energy High-Protein Diet #1 —
8400 kJ (2000 kcal), 77 g Protein

			Energy		
Meal	Food Item	Amount	kJ	kcal	Protein (g)
Breakfast	Whole milk	250 mL (1 cup)	672	160	8
	Orange juice	125 mL ($\frac{1}{2}$ cup)	231	55	1
	Whole-wheat toast with	2 slices	512	122	4
	Butter	15 mL (1 tbsp)	454	108	0
	Poached egg	1 medium	336	80	6
Lunch	Carrot sticks	5 sticks	84	20	0
	Sandwich:				
	Whole-wheat bread	2 slices	512	122	4
	Roast beef	60 g (2 oz)	567	135	14
	Butter	10 mL (2 tsp)	302	72	0
	Mayonnaise	10 mL (2 tsp)	286	68	0
	Pear	1 medium	420	100	1
Snack	Apple juice	125 mL ($\frac{1}{2}$ cup)	256	61	0.5
Evening meal	Whole milk	250 mL (1 cup)	672	160	8
	Broiled salmon	90 g (3 oz)	700	167	22
	Boiled green peas with	125 mL ($\frac{1}{2}$ cup)	298	71	4
	Butter	5 mL (1 tsp)	150	36	0
	Mashed potatoes with	125 mL ($\frac{1}{2}$ cup)	294	70	2
	Butter	5 mL (1 tsp)	150	36	0
	Baked apple with	1 medium	335	80	1
	Brown sugar	15 mL (1 tbsp)	143	34	0
	Butter	15 mL (1 tbsp)	450	108	0
Snack	Peanut butter cookies	2 medium	517	123	2
Total			8345	1988	77

DIARRHEA AND IBD

Diarrhea can be defined as an increased frequency and/or looseness of bowel movements from usual bowel habits. For many individuals with IBD, diarrhea is synonymous with the initiation of the disease, often being the most common initial complaint that stimulates the seeking of medical advice. Diarrhea often continues to be the most common long-term symptom of the disease, with the frequency

Sample High-Energy High-Protein Diet #2 —
10500 kJ (2500 kcal), 93 g Protein

Meal	Food Item	Amount	Energy kJ	Energy kcal	Protein (g)
Breakfast	Whole milk	250 mL (1 cup)	672	160	8
	Orange juice	125 mL ($\frac{1}{2}$ cup)	231	55	1
	Whole-wheat toast	2 slices	512	122	4
	with Butter	15 mL (1 tbsp)	454	108	0
	Poached egg	1 medium	336	80	6
Snack	Apple juice	250 mL (1 cup)	512	122	1
Lunch	Whole milk	125 mL ($\frac{1}{2}$ cup)	336	80	4
	Carrot sticks	5 sticks	84	20	0
	Sandwich:				
	Whole-wheat bread	2 slices	512	122	4
	Roast beef	60 g (2 oz)	567	135	14
	Butter	10 mL (2 tsp)	302	72	0
	Mayonnaise	10 mL (2 tsp)	286	68	0
	Pear	1 medium	420	100	1
Snack	Baked custard	125 mL ($\frac{1}{2}$ cup)	676	161	8
Evening meal	Whole milk	250 mL (1 cup)	672	160	8
	Broiled salmon	90 g (3 oz)	701	167	22
	Boiled green peas	125 mL ($\frac{1}{2}$ cup)	298	71	4
	with Butter	5 mL (1 tsp)	150	36	0
	Mashed potatoes	125 mL ($\frac{1}{2}$ cup)	294	70	2
	with Butter	5 mL (1 tsp)	150	36	0
	Apple pie (two-crust)	$\frac{1}{6}$ standard pie	1697	404	3
Snack	Peanut butter cookies	3 medium	773	184	3
Total			10635	2533	93

of stools ranging from 3 to 30 bowel movements per day. Whether a short-term complaint or a long-term problem, IBD associated diarrhea is one of the more embarrassing and conspicuous symptoms of the disease. From a social perspective, diarrhea can significantly interfere with daily life, as time must be spent looking for and sitting in washrooms, or spent worrying about possible "accidents." From a nutritional perspective, diarrhea can cause severe deficiencies because significant

Sample High-Energy High-Protein Diet #3 —
12600 kJ (3000 kcal), 107 g Protein

Meal	Food Item	Amount	Energy kJ	kcal	Protein (g)
Breakfast	Whole milk	250 mL (1 cup)	672	160	8
	Orange juice	125 mL ($\frac{1}{2}$ cup)	231	55	1
	Whole-wheat toast with	2 slices	512	122	4
	Butter	15 mL (1 tbsp)	454	108	0
	Poached egg	1 medium	336	80	6
Snack	Vanilla milk shake	250 mL (1 cup)	1050	250	8
Lunch	Whole milk	250 mL (1 cup)	672	160	8
	Carrot sticks	5 sticks	84	20	0
	Sandwich:				
	Whole-wheat bread	2 slices	512	122	4
	Roast beef	60 g (2 oz)	567	135	14
	Butter	15 mL (1 tbsp)	454	108	0
	Mayonnaise	10 mL (2 tsp)	286	68	0
	Pear	1 medium	420	100	1
Snack	Baked custard	125 mL ($\frac{1}{2}$ cup)	676	161	8
Evening meal	Whole milk	250 mL (1 cup)	672	160	8
	Fried salmon with	90 g (3 oz)	853	203	22
	White sauce	50 mL ($\frac{1}{4}$ cup)	462	110	2
	Boiled green peas with	125 mL ($\frac{1}{2}$ cup)	298	71	4
	Butter	5 mL (1 tsp)	150	36	0
	Mashed potatoes with	125 mL ($\frac{1}{2}$ cup)	294	70	2
	Butter	5 mL (tsp)	150	36	0
	Apple pie (two-crust)	$\frac{1}{6}$ standard pie	1697	404	3
Snack	Peanut butter cookies	3 medium	773	184	3
	Apple juice	125 mL ($\frac{1}{2}$ cup)	256	61	0.5
Total			12530	2984	106.5

amounts of fluid and nutrients, such as potassium and sodium, may be lost in the diarrhea fluid. The absorption of vitamins, protein, fat, and carbohydrate may also be impaired. Nutrition can be further hampered as individuals alter their diet by avoiding fruits, vegetables, and whole grains in an attempt to control diarrhea. This dietary manipulation frequently results in an unbalanced nutrient intake which

Sample High-Energy High-Protein Diet #4—
14700 kJ (3500 kcal), 115 g Protein

Meal	Food Item	Amount	Energy kJ	kcal	Protein (g)
Breakfast	Whole milk	250 mL (1 cup)	672	160	8
	Orange juice	125 mL ($\frac{1}{2}$ cup)	231	55	1
	Whole-wheat toast with	2 slices	512	122	4
	Butter	15 mL (1 tbsp)	454	108	0
	Peanut butter	15 mL (1 tbsp)	399	95	5
	Jelly	15 mL (1 tbsp)	218	52	0
	Fried egg	1 medium	487	116	6
Snack	Vanilla milk shake	250 mL (1 cup)	1050	250	8
Lunch	Whole milk	250 mL (1 cup)	672	160	8
	Carrot sticks with	5 sticks	84	20	0
	Mayonnaise	15 mL (1 tbsp)	429	102	0
	Sandwich:				
	Whole-wheat bread	2 slices	512	122	4
	Roast beef	60 g (2 oz)	567	135	14
	Butter	15 mL (1 tbsp)	454	108	0
	Mayonnaise	15 mL (1 tbsp)	428	102	0
	Pear	1 medium	420	100	1
Snack	Eggnog	250 mL (1 cup)	1575	375	10
Evening meal	Whole milk	250 mL (1 cup)	672	160	8
	Fried salmon with	90 g (3 oz)	853	203	22
	White sauce	50 mL ($\frac{1}{4}$ cup)	462	110	2
	Boiled green peas with	125 mL ($\frac{1}{2}$ cup)	298	71	4
	Butter	5 mL (1 tsp)	150	36	0
	Mashed potato with	125 mL ($\frac{1}{2}$ cup)	294	70	2
	Butter	5 mL (1 tsp)	150	36	0
	Apple pie	$\frac{1}{6}$ standard pie	1697	404	3
Snack	Peanut butter cookies	3 medium	773	184	3
	Apple juice	125 mL ($\frac{1}{2}$ cup)	256	61	0.5
Total			14770	3517	114.5

further compounds the adverse nutritional effects of the diarrhea. The most extreme practice—fasting during the day in order to avoid bowel movements—significantly impairs nutritional intake.

Because there are many contributing factors to diarrhea, it is important that the cause of the diarrhea be completely investigated. Diarrhea in IBD can reflect active disease, bile salt malabsorption, malabsorption of lactose or fat, bacterial overgrowth, or a completely unrelated cause, such as food poisoning. The treatment of each is different. If it is determined that the diarrhea is caused by active disease, medical management will be necessary. If investigation proves the diarrhea to be caused by lactose intolerance, a lactose-restricted diet will be required. Similarly, in Crohn's disease, if the small bowel has been extensively resected, resulting in fat malabsorption, a restricted-fat diet may be necessary to reduce the diarrhea and the associated malabsorption of nutrients. In Crohn's disease, short resections of the terminal ileum may result in diarrhea caused by bile salt wasting. The use of a bile salt binder, such as cholestyramine, is often helpful in binding the bile salts and thus in resolving the diarrhea. Bacterial overgrowth, which may occur in

---

DIARRHEA—GENERAL GUIDELINES

If you are experiencing diarrhea, the following guidelines may be helpful. You may wish to try some or all of the suggestions. Emphasis is placed on working with your physician to determine the cause of the diarrhea and receiving the proper treatment. Use the food guides to make wise food choices and to ensure a well-balanced intake. If the source of the diarrhea can be helped by nutrition intervention, such as lactose intolerance, you should seek the advice of a registered dietitian.

- Avoid caffeine.
- Reduce fiber intake.
- Reduce the amount of lactose in the diet.
- Drink plenty of clear fluids, at least 2000 mL (8 cups) per day. If you cannot tolerate them at full strength, dilute juices by adding water.
- Ensure a good intake of potassium.
- Ensure a good intake of sodium. Be liberal with the use of salt and such liquids as broth and bouillon.
- Reduce fatty foods and highly spiced foods in your diet.
- Choose smaller meals and eat frequently.
- Take a well-balanced multivitamin and mineral supplement. Refer to the section on vitamin and mineral supplements for further guidance.

Crohn's disease as a result of a fistula (an abnormal communication between two body surfaces or cavities) or stricture in the small intestine will require medical management to resolve the diarrhea. Diarrhea is a complex symptom that may or may not reflect disease activity. It can play havoc with medical, nutritional, and social aspects of daily life and requires prompt and thorough attention. If diarrhea is a problem for you, you should seek medical advice.

CAFFEINE INTAKE AND IBD

Caffeine is present naturally in tea, coffee, chocolate, and kola nuts. For many individuals, beverages account for most of the caffeine consumed in the diet, with smaller amounts obtained from chocolate bars, chocolate flavored foods, and drugs. Once consumed, almost all of the available caffeine is rapidly absorbed, resulting in maximum effects within 45 to 60 minutes. Caffeine produces a variety of physiologic effects. With moderate intakes of 300 to 700 mg, equivalent to three to seven cups of coffee, it stimulates the central nervous system, enlarges the blood vessels, increases stomach acid secretion, speeds up the heart rate, and causes the kidneys to increase urine output. Heavy caffeine intake, defined as more than 700 mg per day, equivalent to more than seven cups of coffee per day, may produce symptoms of irritability, difficulty in sleeping, nervousness, stomach irritation, and diarrhea. Keep in mind that the amount of caffeine to produce adverse effects varies between individuals. The general recommendation for all adults is to limit caffeine from all sources to below approximately 300 mg per day. This is equivalent to 3 to 4 cups of coffee per day. In individuals with IBD, caffeine intake should be greatly reduced, and eliminated if diarrhea is present.

REDUCING CAFFEINE—GENERAL GUIDELINES

- Eliminate caffeine-containing beverages and replace with decaffeinated coffee, weak tea, caffeine-free herbal teas, caffeine-free coffee substitutes, or caffeine-free carbonated beverages, such as gingerale.
- Choose sweets that do not contain chocolate, such as vanilla pudding rather than chocolate pudding.
- Replace regular chocolate with carob, a caffeine-free chocolate substitute. Carob can be used in recipes in place of chocolate, for example, in cookies instead of chocolate chips.

ILEOSTOMY FOR IBD

An ileostomy is a surgically created opening from the surface of the body into the ileum. The opening, about the size of a nickel, is called the stoma. The purpose of an ileostomy is to allow for the elimination of fecal material when the colon, and possibly some of the ileum, has been surgically removed. In IBD, an ileostomy is usually the consequence of a colectomy (the surgical excision of the colon). In the immediate postoperative period, ileostomy output may be very watery and excessive in volume, possibly 2000 mL (8 cups) per day. It is important to ensure that fluid and electrolyte balance is maintained. Over time, approximately two weeks, the body should adapt and the ileostomy output thicken and reduce to approximately 500 mL (2 cups) per day. Because the colon is no longer present to aid in the absorption of fluid, a normal ileostomy output generally continues to be more watery than normal stool. Once adaptation has occurred, an ileostomy does not negatively affect nutrition since absorption of macronutrients and micronutrients is not altered. If a significant amount of the ileum has been removed, vitamin B_{12} supplementation may be required. The food guides should be followed to ensure a well-balanced intake of the essential nutrients. Complications may arise with ileostomies and can often be addressed by dietary modification. Such problems include gas, odor, diarrhea, blockage, and kidney stone formation.

Gas

Gas production may result in abdominal discomfort and distention of the collecting pouch, causing it to accidentally dislodge. If flatus (gas formed in the digestive tract) is a problem, it may be related to aerophagia (habitual air swallowing). To limit aerophagia, eat slowly, chew with the mouth closed, avoid gulping food, and avoid drinking from a straw. Foods such as carbonated beverages and beer should also be avoided. Certain fruits and vegetables may be excessively gassy for some individuals. Individual intolerances can be determined by trial and error. If you are having problems with gas, it may be beneficial to omit certain foods, as listed below, for a short period of time and add them back into the diet one by one to assess tolerance. Keep in mind that an overly restricted diet is not encouraged. Most individuals with an ileostomy tolerate all foods well.

GAS-PRODUCING VEGETABLES

Beans—lima, kidney, navy
Rutabagas
Brussels sprouts
Cabbage
Green peppers

Corn
Onions
Turnips
Peas, dried
Cauliflower
Broccoli
Soybeans
Cucumber

GAS-PRODUCING FRUIT

Apples
Avocados
Melons—watermelon, honeydew, cantaloupe

Odor

Although the odor of the ileostomy fluid can be related to many causes, food may be a contributor. Not all individuals are affected by the same foodstuffs. However, certain foods have been identified as potential odor causers. If odor is a concern, it may be helpful to eliminate the following foods and add them back into the diet one by one to identify the problem foods. Once you identify them, eliminate these foods from the diet.

ODOR-CAUSING FOODS

Asparagus
Corn
Cabbage
Fish
Highly spiced foods
Beer
Dried beans
Onions
Eggs

Diarrhea

Normal ileostomy output is 500 mL (2 cups) per day, although this varies among individuals. If output increases significantly, it is important to prevent dehydration. Drink plenty of fluids, at least 2000 mL (8 cups) per day; replace sodium losses by adding salt freely in the diet; and ensure a good intake of potassium-rich foods, such as orange juice and tomato juice. Laxative foods such as prunes, prune juice, figs, and licorice should be avoided. Refer to pages 77–82 for further information on diarrhea.

Blockage

Foods may get caught in the ileum at the point where it narrows at the wall of the abdomen. To prevent such blockage, it is wise to chew foods well, to avoid foods that tend to absorb water and swell such as dried fruits and popcorn, and to avoid very fibrous foods, such as celery, rhubarb, pineapple, and seeds.

Kidney Stones

Increased water loss through the ileostomy results in the production of concentrated urine. This concentration of urine increases the risk of uric acid stones forming in the kidney. Drink plenty of fluids each day to ensure a good flow of urine and minimize the chance of kidney stone formation.

If you have any concerns about your ileostomy, you should to contact your physician. Often an appointment can be arranged with an enterstomal therapy nurse (a nurse specializing in the care of stomata). Any concerns regarding diet should be discussed with your physician and registered dietitian.

4

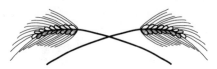

Nutrient Needs in Growth

THE CHILD WITH IBD

IBD afflicts persons of all ages, including the very young, and is associated with a significant incidence of malnutrition. In the young, malnutrition resulting from IBD may be particularly detrimental because the associated failure of growth and development may not be completely reversible, and the physical and emotional side effects last a lifetime. In many situations, it is a failure of growth and development that is the first symptom of IBD and the stimulus to seek medical attention. The factors contributing to malnutrition in the child are the same as for the adult, with a poor dietary intake often being the major contributor. Poor dietary intake can be the result of a general disinterest in food when feeling unwell, a fear of precipitating pain or diarrhea, the adherence to a prescribed overly restrictive diet, or an inability to consume adequate amounts of food when nausea and vomiting are present. Increased losses of nutrients because of malabsorption superimposed on the increased needs of the child with active disease, drugs, and growth can all contribute to malnutrition. Although malnutrition is not solely responsible for the growth failure that can accompany IBD, it is a factor that sometimes is overlooked.

In young patients with Crohn's disease, attempts to prevent or correct growth failure by providing alternate or additional nutrition are frequently initiated. As with adults, the provision of nutrients to children via parenteral nutrition (the delivery of nutrients to the body through a vein) is reserved for very specific situations. The delivery of nutrition through a small flexible tube is more commonly prescribed when possible. The development of special predigested commercial nutritional products, referred to as elemental products, delivered into the stomach by a small feeding tube has allowed for bowel rest and the provision of nutrition. In many situations, all nutritional requirements are provided to the child during the night. This practice allows the child the freedom during the day to attend school and to participate in other activities. If bowel rest is required, little or no other food or fluid is allowed. Refer to the section entitled "Supplemental Nutrition" for further information.

In children with IBD, protein-energy malnutrition is found in association with deficiencies of various vitamins and minerals. The contributory factors are similar to those of adults, with a poor dietary intake being the most important determinant. It is essential that the diet be as unrestricted and as tasty as possible to promote a well-balanced intake. Lactose intolerance is not any more prevalent in children with IBD than in the general population, and it is unnecessary to restrict milk and milk products in children with IBD unless lactose intolerance has been identified. For many children, milk is a major contributor of energy and protein and should not be unnecessarily restricted. Refer to the section on dietary modifications for further discussion on lactose intolerance. Additional restrictions, such as restricted-fiber diets, restricted-fat diets, and the avoidance of spices should not be followed unnecessarily. Unless otherwise instructed by your physician and registered dietitian, an appetizing, well-balanced diet as outlined in the food guides is the best method of caring for all children with IBD.

Although the practice of including daily a well-balanced children's multivitamin and mineral supplement is not dangerous, it should never be considered a replacement for good eating habits. The ingestion of large amounts of nutrients obtained from high-potency supplements is a potentially dangerous practice since it can easily lead to toxicity. A supplement should only be provided to the child with IBD on the recommendation of your physician and with a thorough discussion of its use. Keep in mind that eating habits are developed very early in life. Therefore, for the child with a chronic disease so often associated with malnutrition, it is essential that good eating habits be taught. If your child is not eating well, if you are unsure what constitutes a well-balanced diet, or if your child is required to follow a special diet, it is recommended that you seek advice from your physician and registered dietitian.

**GENERAL GUIDELINES AND TIPS FOR FEEDING
CHILDREN WITH IBD**

- Use the food guides as an outline to ensure a well-balanced intake, but increase the number of servings from the milk group. Children under the age of 9 require two to three servings per day. Children 9 to 12 require three or more servings per day. Teenagers require four servings per day.
- If younger children find the portion sizes, as outlined by the food guides, too large, provide smaller, more frequent meals.
- Do not restrict milk, fiber, fat, or spices in the diet unless advised to do so by your physician and registered dietitian. If dietary restrictions are recommended, ensure that you receive nutrition counseling from a dietitian on how to provide a well-balanced diet. Refer to the corresponding sections in the text to obtain additional information on dietary modification.
- Empty-calorie foods, such as sweets and high-fat snack foods, commonly referred to as "junk food," are a part of most young people's lifestyle and socialization. These foods are allowed in reasonable amounts if nutritional needs are being met as outlined by the food guides.
- Do not use food as a reward for good behavior or punishment for poor behavior. Children need to understand why food and nutrition are important to their bodies.
- If appetite is poor, provide smaller portions of foods more frequently, cater to food likes, reduce bulk by concentrating energy (for example, provide whole milk instead of 2 percent), and provide appetizing meals and snacks in a relaxed atmosphere.

PREGNANCY

Pregnancy is not generally discouraged in individuals with IBD. With proper care, the pregnant woman with IBD can have a normal pregnancy and deliver a healthy child. However, pregnancy, like childhood, is a time of growth, and nutritional intake must be adjusted to meet the increased requirements for a healthy baby. Pregnant women with IBD must pay particular attention to their diets, as IBD is associated with an increased risk of malnutrition. Active IBD associated with nausea, vomiting, or diarrhea, malabsorption of nutrients caused by active disease or extensive small bowel resection, drug-nutrient interactions, and a malnourished state prior to pregnancy may adversely affect nutritional status during pregnancy. These problems may increase nutrient requirements, interfere with nutrient intake, or negatively affect the absorption of nutrients. In general, the dietary guidelines for pregnant women with IBD are the same as for any pregnant woman. The consumption of a well-balanced diet, as outlined in the food guides, is essential to provide for the nutrition needs of the mother and the rapidly growing fetus. If IBD is active, if malabsorption is present, or if certain drugs are required, the diet may require modification. In general, however, a well-balanced diet is encouraged, with as little restriction as possible.

During pregnancy, the nutritional requirement for many nutrients increases. The nutrients that are required in the largest increased amounts include protein, iron, calcium, vitamin D, and folic acid. Energy needs are also increased.

Energy

Energy needs increase in pregnancy in order to provide for the building and maintenance of new tissue and to provide the extra energy required to move around a larger body. During pregnancy, a total weight gain of 11 to 14 kg (25 to 30 lbs) is suggested. The recommended range of weight gain during pregnancy is to some extent related to pre-pregnancy weight. For individuals who are underweight at the beginning of their pregnancy, a greater weight gain is encouraged. The weight gain during pregnancy should be gradual, with the greatest gain occurring in the second half of pregnancy. In Canada, the RNI for pregnant women to provide for weight gain is an extra daily intake of 420 kJ (100 kcal) in the first trimester (a period of three months) and 1250 kJ (300 kcal) in the second and third trimesters. In the United States, the RDA for pregnant women is similar. These increased energy needs can be met easily by increasing the number of servings from the various food groups. Individuals with IBD who are underweight should adjust their diets to provide for greater weight gain. Refer to the section on dietary modifications for practical tips to aid weight gain.

Protein

Protein needs increase in pregnancy to provide for tissue synthesis of mother and fetus. For the mother, such tissue includes the placenta, breasts, and uterus, and proteins in the blood. As the pregnancy progresses, the need for protein increases. In Canada, the recommended additional daily protein intake for women in the first trimester is 5 g, during the second trimester 15 g, and for the third trimester 24 g. In the United States, the additional protein recommendation is 10 g per day for the duration of the pregnancy. These increased needs can be met by increasing the number of servings from protein-rich food groups, such as the milk and meat/alternate groups. Individuals with IBD who have active disease or who are on steroid medications need additional protein to overcome the associated increased losses with disease and steroid medications. Refer to the section on dietary modifications for advice on a high-protein diet.

Iron

The need for iron increases significantly during pregnancy to provide for an increased blood volume and to ensure adequate body supplies for both mother and developing fetus. If adequate iron is not provided, the mother will develop iron deficiency because the fetus will preferentially receive the iron. Iron-deficiency anemia during pregnancy also reduces the iron stores in the baby. In the United States, the RDA for pregnant adult women suggests that the increased requirement cannot be met by diet alone and that supplementation of 30 to 60 mg per day in the form of iron salts is required to prevent iron deficiency. In Canada, the RNI for pregnant women has been established as an extra 5 mg per day in the second trimester and 10 mg per day in the third trimester. The body adapts to the increased need for this nutrient by increasing its absorption in the intestine. Even so, it is most important that iron-rich food choices be eaten on a daily basis to ensure an adequate intake. Individuals with IBD who have iron-deficiency anemia prior to pregnancy will most often require a supplement. This does not, however, preclude the consumption of an iron-rich diet. Refer to the section on dietary modifications for practical advice on improving iron intake.

Calcium

Calcium is required in larger amounts in pregnancy to provide for the development of the skeletal system of the fetus. Most of the deposition of the calcium takes place in the second half of pregnancy. In the United States, the RDA recommends an extra 400 mg of calcium per day to meet these increased needs. In Canada, the RNI has been established as 500 mg per day for pregnant adult females. Increased calcium needs can easily be met by increasing the number of servings from the milk group. A calcium supplement may be required in individuals with severe lactose intolerance. Individuals on steroid medications will require a higher calcium intake to offset the effects of the drugs. Refer to the dietary modifications section for advice on calcium-rich food choices.

Vitamin D

Because this nutrient aids in the absorption of calcium, the requirement for vitamin D also increases in pregnancy. In the United States, the RDA is increased by 5 μg per day. In Canada, the requirement has been established at an additional 2.5 μg per day. The increased requirement for vitamin D can be easily met by consuming extra servings of vitamin-D-fortified milk. This will increase the intake of both vitamin D and calcium.

Folic Acid

This nutrient is required in greater amounts during pregnancy, owing to its role as an essential component of blood. During pregnancy the blood volume of the mother increases, and that of the fetus must be developed. A deficiency of folic acid during pregnancy has been noted in a significant number of pregnant females, and some health care professionals recommend routine supplementation of all pregnant females. For individuals with IBD on a highly restrictive fiber diet or those taking sulfasalazine, or both, supplementation may be necessary to prevent deficiency. In the United States the RDA for pregnant adult women has been established as an additional 220 μg per day. In Canada the RNI has been set at an additional 200 μg per day. A diet rich in food sources of folic acid, such as spinach and other greens, as well as liver, is encouraged. Refer to the section entitled "Key Nutrients in Detail" for further information on folic acid.

If you are pregnant, you should seek further nutritional advice from your physician and registered dietitian. This is especially important if you are underweight, if your disease is active, or if you are following a restrictive diet.

GENERAL DIETARY GUIDELINES FOR PREGNANCY

In order to meet the increased nutritional needs associated with pregnancy, the number of servings and/or the serving size from each food group should be increased. More specifically:

- The number of servings from the milk group should be increased to three to four servings per day.
- Two servings from the meat/alternate group are to be consumed daily.
- An egg should be included in the diet daily or at least three or four times per week.
- An emphasis is placed on whole grains as a source of nutrients including fiber.
- The diet should include one to two servings of dark green leafy vegetables daily.
- One to two servings of vitamin-C-rich fruits or juice should be included in the diet daily.
- Caffeine should be consumed in moderation only.
- Alcohol should not be consumed.
- Salt intake should not be restricted.
- Vitamin and mineral supplements are not to be taken in excess because they may be hazardous to the fetus.

5

Supplemental Nutrition

VITAMIN AND MINERAL SUPPLEMENTS

Vitamin and mineral supplements should never be viewed as an alternative to a well-balanced diet. As supplements, they should complement dietary intake. Unfortunately, the practice of taking large amounts of vitamins and minerals has dramatically increased over the past decade. Many individuals choose to take supplements not only as insurance against nutrient deficiency, but also to obtain therapeutic effects. The promoted benefits from supplement use range from the prevention and cure of specific diseases to increased athletic fitness and improved interpersonal relationships. No scientific data exist to support such claims.

It is very difficult to consume excessive amounts of a vitamin or mineral from the diet, but surprisingly easy to do with a supplement. Many people believe that if a little is good, then a lot is better. The danger of excessive supplementation of the diet with large amounts of vitamins and minerals involves the potential for the development of toxicities. Refer to the specific vitamin or mineral in the section entitled "Key Nutrients in Detail" for further information regarding potential toxicities. The adverse effects of large doses of fat-soluble vitamins are well known and documented. Side effects of overingestion of vitamins A and D range from headache and dizziness to liver damage and coma (a state of abnormal unconsciousness). Adverse effects have also been reported with several of the water-soluble vitamins. For example, an excessive intake of vitamin C has been known to contribute to the development of kidney stones in susceptible individuals. In addition to a direct toxicity, an excessive intake of one nutrient may interfere with the absorption and utilization of another nutrient. For example, excessive zinc intake interferes with copper absorption.

Although supplements should never be used without professional advice, preparations with quantities in excess of normal requirements are available and may be required in specific situations. For example, folic acid supplementation may be required with prolonged use of the drug sulfasalazine; vitamins A and D may be required in chronic fat malabsorption or with long-term use of the drug cholestyramine; or magnesium supplementation may be necessary in an individual who has had significant small bowel resection and excessive stool output.

In IBD, multivitamin and mineral supplements should be taken only when needs cannot be met by a well-balanced diet. If you require a standard multivitamin and mineral preparation to supplement a temporarily restricted diet such as a clear fluid, full fluid, or restricted-fiber diet, use the following table to choose a supplement that is similar to the RNI or RDA. "Natural" vitamin and mineral supplements are not superior to synthetic brands; they are utilized similarly by the body. A registered dietitian can often be helpful in suggesting a well-balanced multivitamin and mineral supplement. When selecting such a supplement, choose one that is similar to the RNI* or RDA* as noted below.

Thiamin	1.1–1.5 mg	Vitamin A	800–1000 RE
Niacin	15–20 mg or NE	Vitamin D	2.5–10μg / 100–400 IU
Riboflavin	1.1–1.7 mg	Vitamin E	7–10 mg
Vitamin B$_6$	1.5–2 mg	Calcium	700–1200 mg
Folate	180–200 μg	Magnesium	200–350 mg
Vitamin B$_{12}$	1–2 μg	Iron	9–15 mg
Vitamin C	30–60 mg	Zinc	9–15 mg

* Based on a range for males and females aged 19 to 24 years.

COMMERCIAL ORAL NUTRITIONAL SUPPLEMENTS

Nutritional supplementation can be achieved through the use of commercially available oral products. The more common, readily available supplements are marketed as meal replacement products and may be recommended to individuals with IBD as a means of providing a higher energy and protein intake. When consumed with meals or as between-meal snacks on a regular basis, these products do result in weight gain. Besides convenience and the absence of milk for those with lactose intolerance, little is to be gained with the more common supplements over a homemade milk shake. The vanilla milk shake recipe in the recipe section is similar in energy and protein content to most of the standard products, but is one-quarter the cost. Generally increased energy and protein needs can be met with milk shakes between meals and simple dietary manipulation as outlined in the sections entitled "High-Energy Diet" and "High-Protein Diet."

Commercial nutritional supplements can be helpful in active disease when cramping, diarrhea, poor appetite, and a lack of energy interfere with the attainment of a well-balanced diet. Standard low-fiber, nutritionally complete, lactose-free products can be taken as the sole source of nutrition to help maintain nutritional status until standard fluids and solids can be reintroduced into the diet. (Nutritionally complete means that, within a given volume, a food contains adequate nutrients to meet nutritional needs when taken as the sole source of nutrition.) These products are also helpful in complementing a full fluid diet when lactose intolerance is present and milk shakes are not tolerated. If convenience is a key issue, these products are handy to have in the car or purse as a quick and easy between-meal snack when other food or drink is not available.

Many of the commercial oral nutritional supplements are similar in composition, often containing 4.2 kJ (1 kcal) per mL or 1000 kJ (250 kcal) per serving along with a balance of various vitamins and minerals. Generally packaged in ready-to-serve 235 mL (8 oz) cans or boxes, the cost of these products ranges from $1.50 to $3.00, and they are available at most pharmacies and large grocery stores. Various flavors are available, with the most common being vanilla, chocolate, and strawberry. A major difference between the various products is the presence or absence of milk, which is an important consideration for those individuals with lactose intolerance. The following is a partial list of oral commercial supplements. Product availability, cost, and nutrient composition may vary from geographic area to area. Individualized guidance by a registered dietitian is advised to help ensure that you obtain the most appropriate product at the best price.

AVAILABLE PRODUCTS

- Oral Nutritional Supplements: milk-based. These are generally nutritionally complete, low-fiber products, containing 4.2 kJ/mL (1 kcal/mL). The liquid products are usually packaged in ready-to-serve individual serving size cans or boxes. Powdered products are to be mixed with milk. The most common products are available in drug stores and some grocery stores. Examples: Meritene®, Sustacal®.

- Oral Nutritional Supplements: milk-free (lactose-free). These are generally nutritionally complete, low-fiber products, containing 4.2 kJ/mL (1 kcal/mL). They are available in various flavors in drug stores and some grocery stores. Often several flavors are available. The liquid products are usually ready-to-serve and packaged in individual serving size cans or boxes. Examples: Ensure®, Resource®, Nutren1®.
- Oral Nutritional Supplements—Energy Dense: milk-free (lactose-free). These are generally nutritionally complete, low-fiber products, containing 6.3 kJ/mL (1.5 kcal/mL). They are available in drug stores and grocery stores in a range of flavors. The liquid products are often ready-to-serve and packaged in individual serving size cans or boxes. These products are more energy-dense than the above products and are useful when stomach capacity is limited. To obtain the higher energy content, these products are often higher in fat. Examples: Ensure plus®, Resource plus®, Nutren 1.5®.

SPECIAL PRODUCTS

- Clear, lactose-free, low-fat nutritional supplements. For individuals on a clear fluid diet and/or a low-fat diet, the above products may not be appropriate. Special products are available that do not fall into the categories listed above. These products are helpful in enhancing the nutritional value, especially the protein content, of a clear fluid diet, and the energy value of a low-fat diet. They offer an alternative to the "milky" supplements previously listed. The following products are nutritionally complete, low in fiber, and low in fat. They are available in various flavors, as a powder in cartons of single-serving packages, or in multi-serving cans. Examples: Citrotein, Surgical Liquid Diet®(SLD).
- Single-nutrient products. The following products are not nutritionally complete, but instead are a source of carbohydrate only. Available in powder and/or ready-to-use liquid form, these products are to be added to the diet to improve energy intake without increasing volume. They can be added directly to a food or fluid both in a powder or in liquid form, since they readily mix into foods such as mashed potatoes and fluids such as juice or soup. When added to foods or fluids, they do not alter the flavor. These products are helpful additions to a clear fluid diet or a low-fat diet to increase energy value. Examples: Polycose, Caloreen®.
- Elemental nutritional products. Most nutritionally complete commercial products contain whole protein and generous amounts of fat. For individ-

uals with IBD who have a reduced ability to digest and absorb these nutrients and for individuals who require bowel rest, very specialized nutritional products are available. These products contain protein in a predigested form, either as amino acids (the building blocks of protein) or as peptides (short chains of amino acids) and are lower in fat to provide for minimal gut stimulation and stool production. These products are referred to as elemental diets. They may be prescribed for either oral consumption or tube feeding. Because they are specialized, they are costly, not readily available, and should not be taken unless prescribed and monitored by a physician and registered dietitian. Examples: Vital HN®, Vivonex T.E.N.®, Flexical®.

TUBE FEEDING AND PARENTERAL NUTRITION

As much as possible, good nutrition should be provided through a well-balanced diet. Sometimes, despite dedicated efforts by the individual, his or her nutritional state declines. Weight loss and muscle wasting may result, which reduces the energy level and the ability to carry out usual daily activities. In such circumstances, alternative nutritional support may be required. An acceptable method of nutritional supplementation, particularly for Crohn's disease, involves the delivery of a liquid formula directly into the stomach through a small, pliable feeding tube passed through the nasal passage. This route of feeding is referred to as a nasogastric feed. In some instances, the feeding tube may be placed directly into the stomach through the wall of the abdomen. Depending on where the feeding tube enters and where the tip of the tube rests, this type of tube feeding is referred to by different names. For example, if the entry site of the tube is the stomach and the tip is also in the stomach, it is referred to as a gastrostomy tube feed. Providing nutrition through tube feeding may be done on a nightly basis with removal or clamping of the tube each morning to allow the individual the freedom to go about daily activities. Additional foods may or may not be allowed depending on the individual's situation. If bowel rest is desired or if significant malabsorption is present, an elemental product may be prescribed. In many cases a standard tube feeding formula is adequate to meet nutritional needs especially when the goal is to provide extra energy to either prevent weight loss or to promote weight gain. In both situations, nighttime tube feeding often results in weight gain, improved nutrition, and an enhanced sense of well-being.

A second route of providing nutritional support is delivery of nutritional solutions into a vein. Previously referred to as intravenous alimentation, this is more commonly referred to as parenteral nutrition, total parenteral nutrition, or simply TPN. This method provides the necessary nutrients to the body without using the gastrointestinal tract. Like nasogastric tube feeding, parenteral nutrition is often administered at night and stopped in the morning to allow for normal daily activities. Additional food and liquid may or may not be allowed. Parenteral nutrition is much more expensive and hazardous than tube feeding and is limited to very specific situations. Whenever possible, the safest, most beneficial, and least expensive method of providing nutrition is used.

Both tube feeding and parenteral nutrition are common in the hospital setting. Both forms of nutrition support can also be provided outside of the hospital in the home environment. In many cases, the tube feeding or parenteral nutrition is initiated in the hospital and the individual is taught for continued care in the home. If home tube feedings or parenteral nutrition have been prescribed for you, it is important that you work closely with the health care team. This team often includes a physician, nurse, dietitian, and pharmacist. The health care team will work with you to choose the most appropriate product, instruct you on how to prepare and deliver the product, and obtain any supplies you need. The health care team will also advise you as to what you should or should not be eating, and offer advice on aspects of living with home nutrition. Although both tube feeding and parenteral nutrition are safe in experienced hands, neither method is without potential hazard. Every member of the health care team has a specific role to play in ensuring that the nutrition support you receive is safe and beneficial. Because you are the key member of the team, it is important for you to have regular contact with the other team members. You should arrange regular visits with the team and contact them immediately if a problem arises.

6

Food Budgeting

With increasing food costs, it is very important to shop wisely in order to get the most from your food dollar. For some individuals, money spent unwisely may interfere with the ability to purchase and consume a well-balanced diet. In order to ensure that poor eating habits do not arise from inadequate funds, the following list of practical suggestions are included to help you manage your food budget.

BUDGETING TIPS FOR EACH FOOD GROUP

MILK GROUP

- Skim milk powder is often less expensive than fluid milk. Use in place of fluid milk in baked products, puddings, soups, sauces, and so on.
- If you are trying to increase protein and energy intake, skim milk powder is an easy and economical way to achieve this goal. Add to fluid milk to drink and to use in recipes, casseroles, soups, and so on.

BUDGETING—GENERAL GUIDELINES

- Plan your week's menus ahead of time, taking advantage of savings noted in grocery store fliers.
- Remember to plan your menus and shop with the food guides in mind. It is not a savings if good nutrition rules are not followed.
- Be aware of your family's likes and dislikes. It is not a savings if the family will not eat or does not enjoy the food.
- Save and use food discount coupons. Remember to compare brand costs because a discount coupon may not reduce the cost of a particular brand below a competitor's price.
- Always prepare a shopping list before going to the grocery store. This helps prevent impulse buying.
- Limit shopping to once a week, as more frequent shopping leads to impulse buying.
- Never shop on an empty stomach, as this often leads to overshopping.
- Remember that high-priced products are placed at eye level on the shelf of many grocery stores. Bend over and scan the lower shelves and compare cost.
- Generic or house brands are frequently less costly than more highly advertised products. Taste and compare cost.
- Avoid or limit convenience foods, since these are often more expensive because of processing and packaging. This includes T.V. dinners, prepackaged vegetables in sauces, breaded fish or chicken, ready-to-eat-cereals, and so forth.

- Making your own yogurt can be significantly less expensive than purchasing it in the grocery store.
- Buy yogurt in large containers, as it is less expensive than individual serving size containers. If you need it for lunch boxes for work or school, add it to smaller containers.
- Stock up on yogurt when it is on sale. Yogurt keeps very well in the refrigerator for a significant length of time.
- Buy plain yogurt and add your own fruit. This is higher in nutritional value as well as being less expensive.
- Buy cheese in bulk instead of buying prepackaged products, especially presliced or individually wrapped cheese. The more packaging, generally, the more expensive the item. Don't forget to compare cost.
- Stock up on cheese when it is on sale. If you cannot use it within a reasonable length of time, store it in the freezer. Freezing cheese may alter its texture, but is quite acceptable for grating and adding to casseroles, soups, chili, sauces, and so forth.

- Cheese that has hardened in the refrigerator does not have to be thrown out. It makes an acceptable product for grating and adding to soups, sauces, and so on.
- Store food properly so that it does not spoil. Food that spoils and cannot be eaten adds to food costs. Follow these guidelines:
  - Fresh milk should be refrigerated as soon as possible and used within a week.
  - Unrefrigerated milk must be used that day.
  - Store skim milk powder in a cool dry place. It has a shelf life of months.
  - Store cheese in a cool dry place. Once you open it, wrap it in plastic.
  - Soft cheese spoils more readily than hard cheese. Cottage cheese should be eaten within a few days.
  - Hard cheese can be stored for two to three months.

MEAT/ALTERNATE GROUP

- Rather than buying presliced luncheon meats, it is less expensive to cook a beef roast or whole chicken and slice the meat into individual servings for freezing until needed. Meat can be frozen in individual packages or in packages of several servings.
- Buy less expensive cuts of meat, such as a blade steak rather than a T-bone steak, and marinate or use cooking methods that will tenderize. Generally, slow cooking with moist heat will tenderize meat. Another alternative is to freeze meat slightly, slice in very thin strips, and use in stir frying.
- Buy meat in bulk when it is on sale. If it comes in large portion sizes, reduce it to smaller recipe size portions before freezing.
- Use your imagination and experiment with less expensive, less common meats such as heart, tongue, kidney, and so on. Try a chicken liver and vegetable stir fry!
- Generally, chicken and turkey are less expensive than red meats. Choose these meats more often.
- Stock up when you find a good sale on canned fish. It has a long shelf life and is quick and easy for sandwiches, casseroles, and salads. Stretch your food dollar by adding yogurt or mayonnaise, chopped onion, or chopped celery when using it for sandwiches.
- Although convenient, frozen fish that has been breaded or partially cooked is often not a good buy because the extra processing adds to the cost of the product.
- If you are making hamburgers or meatloaf, stretch your food dollar by adding oatmeal or cooked rice to the raw mixture.
- Try to plan one meatless meal per week, for example macaroni and cheese, vegetable chili, vegetable quiche, and so on.

- Dried peas and beans are often less expensive than canned ones are.
- Buying dried beans and peas in large quantities is often cost effective.
- Proper storage is important to retain nutrient value and to prevent spoilage. Follow these guidelines:
    - Raw meat should be stored in the refrigerator as soon as possible after purchase.
    - As a general rule, the larger the piece of meat, the longer it can be stored. Ground meat should be used within one day of purchase. Roasts will keep for two to three days. If you cannot use meat within this time frame, freeze it.
    - Fresh or frozen fish must be handled properly, as it deteriorates quickly. Fish stored in the freezer should be used within three months.
    - Raw and cooked chicken should be used within one to two days. If you do not use it immediately, freeze it.
    - Store dried peas and beans in a cool place.

BREAD/CEREAL GROUP

- Many grocery stores and bakeries sell day-old bread at a significant savings. When possible, buy it in quantity and freeze for future use.
- Dry or stale bread should not be thrown out, but diced for croutons, stuffing, or bread puddings.
- To make bread crumbs, completely dry out stale bread and crush by placing bread in a bag and gently crushing with a rolling pin. Bread crumbs can be used as a meat extender, coating for baked chicken or fish, or topping for casseroles.
- Ready-to-eat cereals, especially the pre-sweetened types are convenient but generally expensive. Hot cereals that need to be prepared such as oatmeal, Cream of Wheat, and Cream of Rice are a better buy.
- Leftover rice can be heated and used as a hot breakfast cereal. Add raisins and top with milk and syrup.
- Plainly shaped pasta is less expensive than pasta cut in fancy shapes such as wheels or bows.
- Plain white or brown rice is a better buy than flavored mixes. To flavor plain rice, cook it in beef or chicken broth or use orange juice in place of water for part of the liquid. Chopped onion, nuts, and even raisins can be added to spice up the flavor.
- When on sale, buy unperishable staples such as rice and flour in large quantities. Make sure, however, that you have adequate storage space.
- As with produce and meats, storage is important. Store breads in a cool, dry place. Store rice, rolled oats, and flour in jars or containers that have tight-fitting lids.

FRUIT/VEGETABLE GROUP

- Buy produce when in-season only. Off-season it will often be much more expensive.
  - Winter—oranges, grapefruit, bananas, root vegetables
  - Summer—most salad vegetables, corn, beans, peaches, cherries, melons
  - Fall—cabbage, broccoli, beets, squash, cauliflower, apples, pears, plums, grapes
  - Spring—rhubarb, lettuce, spinach
- Buy ripe bananas in large quantity when on sale. They can be mashed and used immediately or frozen for future use in such baked items as muffins and breads.
- Cabbage makes an excellent salad and is often less expensive than lettuce.
- Canned and frozen produce is often less expensive than imported fresh produce.
- Buying produce in bulk is often a better buy. It is not a good buy, however, if it is not used quickly enough and it spoils. Buy in bulk, but plan your menu wisely.
- Like bananas, other fruits that are just a bit too ripe for eating plain can be easily used in baked products. If you cannot use them immediately, mash or puree and freeze.
- Canned fruit packed in water is less expensive than that packed in heavy syrup.
- Generally, the smallest vegetables and the largest fruits are the preferred produce and hence often the most expensive. Less preferred produce is just as nutritious but more reasonable in cost.
- Convenience items, such as frozen vegetables in sauce or butter, are much more costly than plain frozen items. Buy plain frozen vegetables and fruits and add your own sauce, butter, or spices.
- Produce is very fragile and must be stored properly to retain freshness and nutritional value. General guidelines are covered in detail in the section on retaining nutritional value.

II

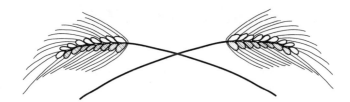

Recipes

The following recipe section has been included to encourage balanced eating habits through practical examples. An *approximated* nutritional analysis has been given for each recipe as a matter of interest and to help you choose those dishes that are good sources of the nutrients you may be seeking. Whenever appropriate, serving suggestions and advice on dietary modifications and restrictions have been stated. A week of menus using some of the recipes is included at the end of the recipe section. Enjoy!

7

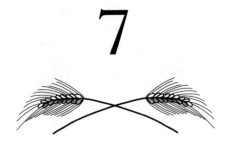

Beverages

ENRICHED MILK

4 servings

Ingredients

| 1000 mL | Whole milk | 4 cups |
| 250 mL | Skim milk powder | 1 cup |

Combine ingredients, mixing well.

Serving Suggestions

Serve in place of regular milk to drink or in any recipe as an easy way to improve energy, protein, and calcium intake.

Nutrients per Serving

Energy	1155 kJ	Vitamin C	5 mg
	275 kcal	Calcium	705 mg
Protein	20 g	Potassium	960 mg
Fat	8.8 g	Iron	0.2 mg
Vitamin A	336 IU	Zinc	2.2 mg
Folacin	29 μg	Fiber	0 g
Vitamin B$_{12}$	2.2μg		

Dietary Modifications

Restricted fat
Replace whole milk with skim milk.

Restrictions

This recipe is not suitable for a restricted-lactose diet.

SHERBET SHAKE

2 servings

Ingredients

250 mL	Skim milk	1 cup
250 mL	Orange sherbet	1 cup
30 mL	Skim milk powder	2 tbsp

Combine ingredients in a blender and whip until smooth.

Serving Suggestions

Serve immediately in a chilled glass.

A refreshing, light, low-fat, high-protein drink.

Nutrients per Serving

Energy	900 kJ	Vitamin C	4 mg
	215 kcal	Calcium	310 mg
Protein	8.3 g	Potassium	456 mg
Fat	2.3 g	Iron	0.2 mg
Vitamin A	365 IU	Zinc	1.5 mg
Folacin	17 μg	Fiber	0 g
Vitamin B$_{12}$	0.9 μg		

Dietary Modifications

High energy
  Replace skim milk with whole milk.

Restrictions

This recipe is not suitable for a restricted-lactose diet.

BANANA-O.J. WHIP

1 large serving

Ingredients

250 mL	Orange juice	1 cup
1 medium	Banana, cut up	

Place ingredients in blender and whip at high speed until smooth.

Serving Suggestions

Pour over ice to chill, and serve immediately.

A refreshing high-potassium breakfast drink or snack.

Nutrients per Serving

Energy	1155 kJ	Vitamin C	115 mg
	275 kcal	Calcium	31 mg
Protein	3 g	Potassium	967 mg
Fat	0.7 g	Iron	0.6 mg
Vitamin A	300 IU	Zinc	0.3 mg
Folacin	140 μg	Fiber	2.4 g
Vitamin B$_{12}$	0 μg		

VANILLA SHAKE

1 serving

Ingredients

250 mL	Enriched milk*	1 cup
125 mL	Vanilla ice cream	$\frac{1}{2}$ cup

Combine all ingredients in a blender, mixing until smooth and frothy.

Serving Suggestions

Serve immediately in a chilled glass.

An excellent high-energy, high-protein addition to a full fluid diet.

Nutrients per Serving

Energy	1825 kJ	Vitamin C	4 mg
	435 kcal	Calcium	705 mg
Protein	19.8 g	Potassium	960 mg
Fat	21.3 g	Iron	0.3 mg
Vitamin A	800 IU	Zinc	2.62 mg
Folacin	27 µg	Fiber	0 g
Vitamin B_{12}	2.2 µg		

Restrictions

This recipe is not suitable for a restricted-lactose or restricted-fat diet.

*Refer to Enriched Milk recipe.

SUPER-STRENGTH SHAKE

2 servings

Ingredients

250 mL	Buttermilk	1 cup
50 mL	Skim milk powder	$\frac{1}{4}$ cup
125 mL	Vanilla ice cream	$\frac{1}{2}$ cup
125 mL	Orange juice	$\frac{1}{2}$ cup
30 mL	Sugar	2 tbsp

Combine all ingredients in a blender, mixing at high speed until smooth.

Serving Suggestions

Serve immediately in a chilled glass.

An excellent nutritious addition to a full fluid diet, and a quick high-calcium breakfast or snack idea.

Nutrients per Serving

Energy	1135 kJ	Vitamin C	28 mg
	270 kcal	Calcium	355 mg
Protein	10.3 g	Potassium	600 mg
Fat	7.5 g	Iron	0.2 mg
Vitamin A	335 IU	Zinc	1.4 mg
Folacin	36 μg	Fiber	0 g
Vitamin B$_{12}$	0.9 μg		

Restrictions

This recipe is not suitable for a restricted-lactose or restricted-fat diet.

MONKEY MAPLESHAKE

1 serving

Ingredients

125 mL	Whole milk	$\frac{1}{2}$ cup
125 mL	Plain yogurt	$\frac{1}{2}$ cup
1 medium	Banana, cut up	
15–30 mL	Maple syrup	1–2 tbsp

Combine all ingredients in a blender, mixing until smooth.

Serving Suggestions

Serve immediately in a chilled glass.

A quick, high-energy, high-protein, calcium-rich breakfast or snack.

Nutrients per Serving

Energy	1300 kJ	Vitamin C	13 mg
	310 kcal	Calcium	326 mg
Protein	9.6 g	Potassium	884 mg
Fat	8.7 g	Iron	0.7 mg
Vitamin A	406 IU	Zinc	1.36 mg
Folacin	37 μg	Fiber	2.2 g
Vitamin B$_{12}$	0.9 μg		

Dietary Modifications

Restricted fat
   Replace whole milk with skim milk.
   Choose low-fat yogurt.

High protein
   Add 30 mL (2 tbsp) skim milk powder.

Restrictions

This recipe is not suitable for a restricted-lactose diet.

FRUITY YOGURT SHAKE

1 serving

Ingredients

250 mL	Plain yogurt	1 cup
30 mL	Skim milk powder	2 tbsp
125 mL	Apple juice	$\frac{1}{2}$ cup
7 mL	Brown sugar	$1\frac{1}{2}$ tsp
1 medium	Banana, cut up	

Combine all ingredients, except banana, in blender. Add banana and whip until smooth.

Serving Suggestions

Serve immediately in a chilled glass.

An excellent light breakfast or snack idea.

Nutrients per Serving

Energy	1635 kJ	Vitamin C	14 mg
	390 kcal	Calcium	500 mg
Protein	15 g	Potassium	1285 mg
Fat	8.6 g	Iron	1.2 mg
Vitamin A	400 IU	Zinc	2.2 mg
Folacin	47 μg	Fiber	2.2 g
Vitamin B$_{12}$	1.5 μg		

Dietary Modifications

Restricted lactose
  Choose yogurt that does not contain added milk solids.
  Do not add skim milk powder.

Restricted fat
  Choose low-fat yogurt.

High energy
  Choose high-fat yogurt.

Restrictions

This recipe may not be suitable if one is significantly lactose intolerant.

BLUEBERRY YOGURT SHAKE

1 serving

Ingredients

250 mL	Whole milk	1 cup
80 mL	Frozen blueberries	$\frac{1}{3}$ cup
180 mL	Blueberry yogurt	$\frac{3}{4}$ cup

Combine all ingredients in blender, mixing until smooth.

Serving Suggestions

Top with more blueberries and serve immediately in a chilled glass.
A delicious high-energy breakfast drink or snack idea.

Nutrients per Serving

Energy	1890 kJ	Vitamin C	4 mg
	450 kcal	Calcium	565 mg
Protein	15 g	Potassium	800 mg
Fat	12 g	Iron	0.6 mg
Vitamin A	445 IU	Zinc	1.7 mg
Folacin	18 μg	Fiber	0.6 g
Vitamin B$_{12}$	1.3 μg		

Dietary Modifications

Restricted lactose
Use milk treated with a commercial lactase enzyme product.
Choose yogurt that does not contain added milk solids.

Restricted fat
Replace whole milk with skim milk.
Choose low-fat yogurt.

High protein
Add 60 mL (4 tbsp) skim milk powder.

Restrictions

This recipe is not suitable for a restricted-fiber diet or a restricted-lactose diet if one is significantly lactose intolerant.

HIGH-PROTEIN NOG

2 servings

Ingredients

500 mL	Enriched milk*	2 cups
1	Egg yolk	
30 mL	Sugar	2 tbsp
2 mL	Vanilla extract	$\frac{1}{2}$ tsp
0.5 mL	Salt	$\frac{1}{8}$ tsp
sprinkle	Nutmeg	

In a saucepan, beat sugar into egg yolk. Stir in remaining ingredients and cook over low heat. Remove from heat when mixture coats spoon.

Serving Suggestions

Can be served hot or cold.

An excellent energy-rich, high-calcium, high-protein addition to a full fluid or regular diet.

Nutrients per Serving

Energy	1405 kJ	Vitamin C	4 mg
	335 kcal	Calcium	640 mg
Protein	19 g	Potassium	855 mg
Fat	11.5 g	Iron	0.7 mg
Vitamin A	490 IU	Zinc	2.28 mg
Folacin	38 μg	Fiber	0 g
Vitamin B$_{12}$	2.3 μg		

Dietary Modifications

Restricted fat
Replace whole milk with skim milk.

Restrictions

This recipe is not suitable for a restricted-lactose diet.

*Refer to Enriched Milk recipe.

TOFU SHAKE

2 servings

Ingredients

125 mL/120 g	Tofu	$\frac{1}{2}$ cup/4 oz
125 mL	Plain yogurt	$\frac{1}{2}$ cup
30 mL	Powdered skim milk	2 tbsp
125 mL	Diced peaches	$\frac{1}{2}$ cup
1 medium	Banana, cut up	
5 mL	Lemon juice	1 tsp
15 mL	Sugar	1 tbsp

Combine all ingredients in a blender, mixing until smooth.

Serving Suggestions

Serve immediately in a chilled glass.

A nutritious fruity breakfast drink or snack.

Nutrients per Serving

Energy	880 kJ	Vitamin C	11 mg
	210 Kcal	Calcium	237 mg
Protein	10.6 g	Potassium	635 mg
Fat	5.2 g	Iron	3.5 mg
Vitamin A	437 IU	Zinc	1.3 mg
Folacin	30 μg	Fiber	2 g
Vitamin B$_{12}$	0.5 μg		

Dietary Modifications

Restricted lactose

Choose yogurt without added milk solids.
Omit skim milk powder.

Restrictions

This recipe is not suitable for a restricted-lactose diet if one is significantly lactose intolerant.

8

Soups and Salads

Borscht

Chicken-Rice Soup

Mulligatawny Soup

Filling Fish Soup

Easy Cheesy Tomato Soup

Cream of Asparagus Soup

Cool and Creamy Carrot Soup

Fresh Salad Delight

Sunshine Salad

Marinated Vegetables

Waldorf Salad

Spinach-Orange Salad

Greek Salad

Spiced Turkey Salad

Cottage Cheese and Fruit Salad

121

BORSCHT

4 servings

Ingredients

250 mL	Beets, shredded	1 cup
250 mL	Carrots, diced	1 cup
125 mL	Onion, chopped	$\frac{1}{2}$ cup
375 mL	Water, salted, boiling	$1\frac{1}{2}$ cups
2	Beef bouillon cubes	
375 mL	Water, boiling	$1\frac{1}{2}$ cups
125 mL	Cabbage, shredded	$\frac{1}{2}$ cup
15 mL	Margarine	1 tbsp
pinch	Pepper	

Cook beets, carrots, and onion uncovered in salted boiling water for 20 to 25 minutes. In a separate bowl, dissolve beef bouillon cubes in boiling water. Add beef bouillon, cabbage, margarine, and pepper to beet mixture, and cook uncovered for an additional 15 minutes.

Serving Suggestions

Serve hot, topped with a dollop of sour cream.

Serve for lunch with roast beef sandwiches, a glass of milk, and cookies.

Nutrients per Serving

Energy	336 kJ	Vitamin C	12 mg
	80 kcal	Calcium	31 mg
Protein	1.9 g	Potassium	287 mg
Fat	3.6 g	Iron	0.7 mg
Vitamin A	10,000 IU	Zinc	0.3 mg
Folacin	32 μg	Fiber	2.1 g
Vitamin B_{12}	0 μg		

Dietary Modifications

Restricted lactose
  Omit sour cream.
Restricted fat
  Reduce margarine to 5 mL (1 tsp).

High energy
  Increase the amount of margarine to 30 mL (2 tbsp) or more.
  Use generous amounts of sour cream.

Restrictions

This recipe is not suitable for a restricted-fiber diet.

CHICKEN-RICE SOUP

6 servings

Ingredients

1.2 L	Chicken broth	5 cups
2	Garlic cloves, crushed	
50 mL	Onion, chopped	$\frac{1}{4}$ cup
50 mL	Carrot, shredded	$\frac{1}{4}$ cup
375 mL	Chicken, cooked, diced	$1\frac{1}{2}$ cups
125 mL	Rice, uncooked	$\frac{1}{2}$ cup
dash	Pepper	
dash	Salt	
pinch	Sage	

Bring broth to simmer. Add all ingredients to broth. Cover and simmer for 20 minutes.

Serving Suggestions

Serve hot for lunch, alone or with sandwiches.

A light meal on days when appetite is poor.

Nutrients per Serving

Energy	630 kJ	Vitamin C	1 mg
	150 kcal	Calcium	14 mg
Protein	12 g	Potassium	130 mg
Fat	3 g	Iron	1 mg
Vitamin A	1100 IU	Zinc	1 mg
Folacin	6 μg	Fiber	0.4 g
Vitamin B$_{12}$	0.1 μg		

Dietary Modifications

Restricted Fiber
   Omit onion.

MULLIGATAWNY SOUP

4 servings

Ingredients

30 mL	Margarine	2 tbsp
125 mL	Chicken, uncooked, diced	$\frac{1}{2}$ cup
1 small	Onion, chopped	
1 medium	Celery stalk, diced	
1 small	Carrot, diced	
1 small	Apple, pared, diced	
30 mL	White flour	2 tbsp
2.5 mL	Curry powder	$\frac{1}{2}$ tsp
750 mL	Chicken broth	3 cups
1 small	Tomato, peeled, chopped	
2.5 mL	Salt	$\frac{1}{2}$ tsp
2.5 mL	Minced parsley	$\frac{1}{2}$ tsp
dash	Pepper	
125 mL	Rice, cooked	$\frac{1}{2}$ cup

In a saucepan melt margarine. Add chicken, onion, celery, carrot, and apple and cook until lightly browned. Add flour and curry powder and mix while slowly stirring in the chicken broth. Add all remaining ingredients except rice and cook covered for 20 minutes. Add rice and heat through.

Serving Suggestions

Serve hot.

Can be served alone as a light lunch or with a sandwich, or with pita bread filled with meat and lettuce.

Nutrients per Serving

Energy	840 kJ	Vitamin C	10 mg
	200 kcal	Calcium	25 mg
Protein	9.2 g	Potassium	265 mg
Fat	10.3 g	Iron	1.1 mg

Vitamin A	4000 IU	Zinc	0.7 mg
Folacin	18 μg	Fiber	2.4 g
Vitamin B$_{12}$	0.1 μg		

Dietary Modifications

Restricted fat
Reduce margarine to 15 mL (1 tbsp).

Restricted fiber
Omit celery.
Omit onion.
Remove skin and seeds from tomato.

High protein
Add additional chicken.

High energy
Increase margarine to 50 mL ($\frac{1}{4}$ cup).

FILLING FISH SOUP

4 servings

Ingredients

350 g	Whitefish fillets, raw	12 oz
15 mL	Margarine	1 tbsp
50 mL	Onion, chopped	$\frac{1}{4}$ cup
1 medium	Carrot, sliced	
1 medium	Potato, diced	
375 mL	Water, boiling	$1\frac{1}{2}$ cups
2 mL	Salt	$\frac{1}{2}$ tsp
2 mL	Pepper	$\frac{1}{2}$ tsp
250 mL	Spinach leaves, raw, chopped	1 cup
250 mL	Whole milk	1 cup

Cut fish into bite-sized pieces. In a saucepan, melt margarine and sauté onions until tender. Add carrot, potato, water, salt, and pepper to pan. Cover and simmer 10 to 15 minutes. Add fish and spinach and cook for 10 more minutes. Add milk and warm, but do not boil, soup.

Serving Suggestions

Serve hot with chunks of buttered French bread.

A hearty protein-rich lunch idea.

Nutrients per Serving

Energy	966 kJ		Vitamin C	12 mg
	230 kcal		Calcium	104 mg
Protein	20 g		Potassium	680 mg
Fat	10 g		Iron	1.1 mg
Vitamin A	6100 IU		Zinc	1.4 mg
Folacin	40 μg		Fiber	1.3 g
Vitamin B_{12}	0.2 μg			

Dietary Modifications

Restricted fat
  Use low-fat milk in place of whole milk.
  Reduce margarine to 5 mL (1 tsp).

Restricted fiber
  Omit spinach.
  Omit onion.

High protein
  Use enriched milk* in place of whole milk.

Restrictions

This recipe is not suitable for a restricted-lactose diet.

* Refer to Enriched Milk recipe.

EASY CHEESY TOMATO SOUP

2 large servings

Ingredients

1 can, 300 g	Tomato soup	$10\frac{3}{4}$ oz
1 soup can	Whole milk	
dash	Pepper	
dash	Worcestershire sauce	
180 mL	Cheddar cheese, shredded	$\frac{3}{4}$ cup

Prepare soup as per can instructions. Add pepper and Worcestershire sauce to taste. Before serving, slowly stir in cheese, mixing well.

Serving Suggestions

Serve hot, garnished with croutons.
A tasty high-energy, high-protein, and calcium-rich soup.
Serve alone or with a salad, open-faced sandwiches, or buttered rolls.

Nutrients per Serving

Energy	1512 kJ	Vitamin C	70 mg
	360 kcal	Calcium	480 mg
Protein	18 g	Potassium	500 mg
Fat	21 g	Iron	2.1 mg
Vitamin A	1300 IU	Zinc	2 mg
Folacin	28 μg	Fiber	0.5 g
Vitamin B$_{12}$	0.8 μg		

Dietary Modifications

Restricted fat
Replace whole milk with skim milk.
Choose a low-fat cheese and reduce to 80 mL ($\frac{1}{3}$ cup).

High Protein
Stir in 50 mL ($\frac{1}{4}$ cup) skim milk powder to soup when heating.
Increase cheese to 250 mL (1 cup).

High energy
Follow high protein suggestions.

Restrictions

This recipe is not suitable for a restricted-lactose diet.

CREAM OF ASPARAGUS SOUP

6 servings

Ingredients

$\frac{1}{2}$ kg	Fresh asparagus	1 lb
2	Chicken bouillon cubes	
250 mL	Water, boiling	1 cup
45 mL	Margarine or butter	3 tbsp
45 mL	White flour	3 tbsp
2.5 mL	Paprika	$\frac{1}{2}$ tsp
2.5 mL	Basil	$\frac{1}{2}$ tsp
2.5 mL	Salt	$\frac{1}{2}$ tsp
750 mL	Whole milk	3 cups

Wash asparagus, remove tips, and cut stalks into 2.5 cm (1 in) pieces. Dissolve bouillon cubes in boiling water. Add asparagus to water and cook until tender (5 to 7 minutes). Remove from heat and blend in a food processor or blender. In a saucepan, melt butter. Blend flour and seasonings into melted butter and slowly stir in milk. Cook and stir until smooth and slightly thickened. Stir in asparagus purée and heat.

Serving Suggestions

Serve hot, alone or garnished with croutons.

An excellent light meal on days when appetite is poor.

Can be served as an appetizer at a main meal.

A delicious way to improve calcium and protein intake.

Nutrients per Serving

Energy	693 kJ	Vitamin C	26 mg
	165 kcal	Calcium	173 mg
Protein	7.2 g	Potassium	438 mg
Fat	10.3 g	Iron	0.8 mg
Vitamin A	1077 IU	Zinc	1 mg
Folacin	98 μg	Fiber	0.9 g
Vitamin B$_{12}$	0.5 μg		

Dietary Modifications

Restricted lactose
Use milk treated with a commercial lactase enzyme product.
Use milk-free margarine if you are highly lactose intolerant.

Restricted fat
Use skim milk in place of whole milk.
Reduce margarine to 30 mL (2 tbsp).

High protein
Add 125 mL ($\frac{1}{2}$ cup) skim milk powder to milk before heating.

High energy
Follow high protein suggestions.
Stir in an additional 15 mL (1 tbsp) margarine to the soup just before serving.

COOL AND CREAMY CARROT SOUP

4 servings

Ingredients

180 mL	Onion, chopped	$\frac{3}{4}$ cup
225 g	Carrot, chopped	$\frac{1}{2}$ lb
15 mL	Butter or margarine	1 tbsp
500 mL	Chicken broth	2 cups
1 mL	Salt	$\frac{1}{4}$ tsp
pinch	Nutmeg	
dash	Pepper	
250 mL	Light cream	1 cup

In a frying pan, sauté onions and carrots in butter until softened. Transfer to a sauce pan; add broth and seasonings. Cover and bring to a boil. Simmer 15 minutes; then remove from heat. Stir in cream. Place in blender and mix until smooth. Chill in refrigerator.

Serving Suggestions

Garnish with parsley and serve chilled with snack crackers.

An excellent vitamin-A-rich light lunch or appetizer.

Nutrients per Serving

Energy	663 kJ	Vitamin C	8 mg
	158 kcal	Calcium	26 mg
Protein	3.7 g	Potassium	305 mg
Fat	11.3 g	Iron	0.4 mg
Vitamin A	16,000 IU	Zinc	0.2 mg
Folacin	14.5 μg	Fiber	1.7 g
Vitamin B$_{12}$	0 μg		

Dietary Modifications

Restricted fiber
　Omit onion.

High protein
　Add 50 mL ($\frac{1}{4}$ cup) skim milk powder to soup while in blender.

High energy
　Follow high protein suggestion.
　Increase butter to 30 mL (2 tbsp).

Restrictions

This recipe is not suitable for a restricted-lactose diet or restricted-fat diet.

FRESH SALAD DELIGHT

4 servings

Ingredients

1 medium	Cucumber, cubed		
1 medium	Tomato, cubed		
1 medium	Avocado, cubed		
80 mL	Mayonnaise	$\frac{1}{3}$ cup	
pinch	Salt		
pinch	Pepper		
pinch	Dill		
500 mL	Alfalfa sprouts	2 cups	

In a bowl, gently combine all ingredients except alfalfa sprouts. Arrange sprouts on four chilled salad plates. Top with vegetable-mayonnaise mixture.

Serving Suggestions

Serve with buttered rolls, cheese wedges, and a glass of milk as a delicious, nutritious light meal.

This salad is a tasty accompaniment to any meal.

Nutrients per Serving

Energy	966 kJ	Vitamin C	15 mg
	230 kcal	Calcium	25 mg
Protein	2.5 g	Potassium	420 mg
Fat	22 g	Iron	1.1 mg
Vitamin A	760 IU	Zinc	0.5 mg
Folacin	48 μg	Fiber	2.4 g
Vitamin B$_{12}$	0 μg		

Dietary Modifications

Restricted lactose
Use pure mayonnaise, not a mayonnaise substitute.

Restrictions

This recipe is not suitable for a restricted-fat diet or restricted-fiber diet.

SUNSHINE SALAD

4 servings

Ingredients

1000 mL	Fresh spinach	4 cups
1 medium	Red apple	
4 slices	Bacon, crisply fried, crumbled	
125 mL	Mandarin orange sections	$\frac{1}{2}$ cup
80 mL	Mayonnaise	$\frac{1}{3}$ cup
20 mL	Orange juice concentrate	4 tsp

Clean spinach, tear into small pieces, and chill. Just before serving, quarter, core, and slice unpared apple into chilled salad bowl. Add bacon, orange slices, and spinach. Toss lightly to combine. Mix mayonnaise with orange juice and spoon over salad.

Serving Suggestions

Serve chilled.

An excellent nutrient-rich appetizer or light lunch.

Raisins may be added to provide additional texture, flavor, and nutrition.

Nutrients per Serving

Energy	987 kJ		Vitamin C	41 mg
	235 kcal		Calcium	68 mg
Protein	4.5 g		Potassium	514 mg
Fat	18.9 g		Iron	2.1 mg
Vitamin A	4315 IU		Zinc	0.6 mg
Folacin	116 μg		Fiber	3.5 g
Vitamin B$_{12}$	0.1 μg			

Dietary Modifications

Restricted lactose

Use pure mayonnaise, not a mayonnaise substitute.

Restricted fat

Do not add bacon.

Replace mayonnaise with low-fat plain yogurt.

Restrictions

This recipe is not suitable for a restricted-fiber diet.

MARINATED VEGETABLES

6 servings

Ingredients

250 mL	Cauliflowerets	1 cup
10	Cherry tomatoes	
250 mL	Broccoli flowerets	1 cup
1 medium	Carrot, cut into strips	
1 medium	Celery stalk, sliced	
250 mL	Mushrooms, whole, raw	1 cup
8	Black olives, pitted, whole	
125 mL	Italian dressing	$\frac{1}{2}$ cup

Prepare vegetables and place in salad bowl. Pour dressing over vegetables and marinate in refrigerator for 24 hours, turning frequently. Drain before serving.

Serving Suggestions

Serve chilled.

An attractive, nutritious party appetizer, side salad, or snack.

Nutrients per Serving

Energy	336 kJ	Vitamin C	27 mg
	80 kcal	Calcium	21 mg
Protein	1.3 g	Potassium	200 mg
Fat	6.9 g	Iron	0.7 mg
Vitamin A	500 IU	Zinc	0.2 mg
Folacin	24 μg	Fiber	0.9 g
Vitamin B$_{12}$	0 μg		

Dietary Modifications

Restricted fat
    Replace regular Italian dressing with a low-fat product.
    Omit olives.

Restrictions

This recipe is not suitable for a restricted-fiber diet.

WALDORF SALAD

6 servings

Ingredients

250 mL	Red apple, diced	1 cup
250 mL	Celery, thinly sliced	1 cup
250 mL	Grape halves, seedless	1 cup
125 mL	Peanuts	$\frac{1}{2}$ cup
50 mL	Raisins	$\frac{1}{4}$ cup
200 mL	Mayonnaise	$\frac{7}{8}$ cup
6 large	Lettuce leaves	

Prepare ingredients and combine with mayonnaise. Arrange a scoop of salad on top of a lettuce leaf.

Serving Suggestions

Serve chilled.

A quick and easy salad to complement any meal.

Nutrients per Serving

Energy	1449 kJ	Vitamin C	5 mg
	345 kcal	Calcium	24 mg
Protein	4.1 g	Potassium	244 mg
Fat	31.2 g	Iron	0.8 mg
Vitamin A	131 IU	Zinc	0.5 mg
Folacin	16 μg	Fiber	2.5 g
Vitamin B$_{12}$	0 μg		

Dietary Modifications

Restricted lactose

Use pure mayonnaise, not a mayonnaise substitute.

Restrictions

This recipe is not suitable for a restricted-fat diet or restricted-fiber diet.

SPINACH-ORANGE SALAD

4 servings

Ingredients

$\frac{1}{2}$ kg	Spinach, raw, fresh	1 lb
125 mL	Mushrooms, raw, fresh, sliced	$\frac{1}{2}$ cup
125 mL	Water chestnuts, sliced, canned	$\frac{1}{2}$ cup
4 medium	Mandarin oranges, sectioned	
80 mL	Raisins	$\frac{1}{3}$ cup
50 mL	Vegetable oil	$\frac{1}{4}$ cup
30 mL	Vinegar	2 tbsp
30 mL	Orange juice	2 tbsp
15 mL	Soy sauce	1 tbsp
pinch	Pepper	
pinch	Salt	

Wash, drain, and remove stems from spinach. Tear spinach into smaller pieces and place in chilled bowl. Add mushrooms, water chestnuts, oranges, and raisins. Combine vegetable oil, vinegar, and remaining ingredients in a jar and shake until well mixed. Pour dressing over salad and toss well.

Serving Suggestions

Serve chilled soon after preparation.

A tasty iron-rich accompaniment to any meal.

Serve with cold meats or cheeses, rolls, and a glass of milk as a light lunch.

Nutrients per Serving

Energy	1071 kJ	Vitamin C	100 mg
	255 kcal	Calcium	187 mg
Protein	6 g	Potassium	1200 mg
Fat	12 g	Iron	4 mg

Vitamin A	9000 IU	Zinc	1 mg
Folacin	250 μg	Fiber	7 g
Vitamin B$_{12}$	0 μg		

Dietary Modifications

Restricted fat
   Reduce oil to 30 mL (2 tbsp) or less.

Restrictions

This recipe is not suitable for a restricted-fiber diet.

GREEK SALAD

4 servings

Ingredients

1000 mL	Lettuce pieces, torn	4 cups
2 medium	Tomatoes, cut into wedges	
1 small	Onion, chopped	
50 mL	Oil and vinegar dressing	$\frac{1}{4}$ cup
80 mL	Feta cheese, crumbled	$\frac{1}{3}$ cup
8	Black olives	
dash	Pepper	

Combine lettuce, tomato, and onion in salad bowl. Add salad dressing and toss well. Top with cheese and olives. Season.

Serving Suggestions

Serve chilled.

More or less olives, onion, and cheese can be added according to taste.

A delicious salad to accompany any meal.

An excellent addition to a traditional Greek meal such as moussaka.

Nutrients per Serving

Energy	567 kJ	Vitamin C	16 mg
	135 kcal	Calcium	95 mg
Protein	3.4 g	Potassium	273 mg
Fat	11 g	Iron	1 mg
Vitamin A	600 IU	Zinc	0.6 mg
Folacin	45 μg	Fiber	1.9 g
Vitamin B$_{12}$	0 μg		

Dietary Modifications

Restricted fat
    Omit olives.
    Choose a low-fat commercial or homemade salad dressing.

Restricted fiber
  Remove skin from tomatoes.
  Omit onion and olives.

High protein
  Add extra cheese.

High energy
  Increase cheese to 125 mL ($\frac{1}{2}$ cup).
  Increase oil to 80 mL ($\frac{1}{3}$ cup).

Restrictions

This recipe is unsuitable for a restricted-lactose diet if cheese is not well tolerated.

SPICED TURKEY SALAD

4 servings

Ingredients

500 mL	Turkey, cooked, diced	2 cups
50 mL	Celery, diced	$\frac{1}{4}$ cup
1 small	Red pepper, chopped	
1 small	Apple, chopped	
50 mL	Peanuts, chopped	$\frac{1}{4}$ cup
50 mL	Raisins	$\frac{1}{4}$ cup
5 mL	Salt	1 tsp
5 mL	Curry powder	1 tsp
dash	Pepper	
180 mL	Mayonnaise	$\frac{3}{4}$ cup
125 mL	Sour cream	$\frac{1}{2}$ cup
4 large	Lettuce leaves	

In a bowl, combine all ingredients except lettuce. Refrigerate mixture until well chilled, about 1 to 2 hours. Arrange lettuce leaves on 4 chilled salad plates. Mound one-quarter of turkey mixture onto each lettuce leaf.

Serving Suggestions

Garnish with parsley, dried coconut, or other suitable garnish.

Turkey salad can be served on alfalfa sprouts in place of lettuce.

Serve as a light lunch accompanied by buttered rolls and milk.

Nutrients per Serving

Energy	2625 kJ	Vitamin C	39 mg
	625 kcal	Calcium	73 mg
Protein	26 g	Potassium	480 mg
Fat	51 g	Iron	2.1 mg

Vitamin A	1435 IU	Zinc	2 mg
Folacin	45 μg	Fiber	2.9 g
Vitamin B$_{12}$	0.3 μg		

Dietary Modifications

Restricted Lactose
  Replace sour cream with pure mayonnaise (not a mayonnaise substitute) or yogurt (no added milk solids).

Restrictions

This recipe is unsuitable for a restricted-fat or restricted-fiber diet. This recipe may be unsuitable on a restricted-lactose diet if yogurt is not well tolerated.

COTTAGE CHEESE AND FRUIT SALAD

2 servings

Ingredients

250 mL	2% cottage cheese	1 cup
2 medium	Lettuce leaves	
1 medium	Peach, sliced	
10 medium	Green grapes, halved	
30 mL	Almonds, sliced	2 tbsp
30 mL	Raisins	2 tbsp

Mound cottage cheese onto lettuce leaves. Arrange peaches and grapes around cottage cheese. Garnish with almonds and raisins.

Serving Suggestions

Serve chilled, accompanied by snack crackers.

An excellent, nutritious light lunch.

Nutrients per Serving

Energy	945 kJ	Vitamin C	9 mg
	225 kcal	Calcium	113 mg
Protein	19 g	Potassium	429 mg
Fat	6 g	Iron	0.9 mg
Vitamin A	414 IU	Zinc	0.8 mg
Folacin	33 μg	Fiber	2.8 g
Vitamin B$_{12}$	0.9 μg		

Dietary Modifications

Restricted fat
   Choose 1% cottage cheese.

Restricted fiber
   Omit raisins and nuts and garnish with parsley.
   Omit grapes and replace with banana slices.
   Remove skin from peach.

High energy
   Choose 4% cottage cheese.

Restrictions

This recipe is not suitable for a restricted-lactose diet.

9

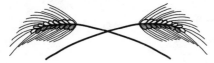

Breads, Cereals, and Grains

Tasty Breakfast Treat

Granola

Oven French Toast

Fruit Pancakes

Cheese Biscuits

Scones

Corn Bread

Dumplings

Fried Rice

Honey-Nut Rice

Orange-Raisin Rice

Barley Bake

TASTY BREAKFAST TREAT

1 serving

Ingredients

1 serving	Hot cereal mix (choose one):	
	Cream of Rice	
	Cream of Wheat	
	Cornmeal	
	Oatmeal	
15–30 mL	Chopped dried fruit:	1–2 tbsp
	Raisins	
	Apricots	
	Peaches	
	Dates	
15–30 mL	Sweetener:	1–2 tbsp
	Sugar (white or brown)	
	Honey	
	Light molasses	
	Maple syrup	
	Preserves, jam, or jelly	

Prepare hot cereal as per package directions for an individual serving, but while heating water to boil, add one or more dried fruits. Top cooked cereal with one or more suggested sweeteners. (Nutrients per Serving table calculated with 125 mL ($\frac{1}{2}$ cup) cream of rice cereal, 15 mL (1 tbsp) raisins, and 15 mL (1 tbsp) honey.

Serving Suggestions

Serve hot topped with milk, cream, or yogurt.

Nutrients per Serving

Energy	609 kJ	Vitamin C	1.4 mg
	145 kcal	Calcium	10.5 mg
Protein	1.3 g	Potassium	100 mg
Fat	0.2 g	Iron	0.4 mg

Vitamin A	0.5 IU	Zinc	0.2 mg
Folacin	4.5 μg	Fiber	0.6 g
Vitamin B$_{12}$	0 μg		

Dietary Modifications

Restricted lactose
Top with milk treated with a commercial enzyme product.

Restricted fat
Top with skim milk or low-fat yogurt.

Restricted fiber
Omit dried fruit and top with fresh banana or peach slices.

High protein
Cook cereal in enriched milk* rather than water.
Top with enriched milk.*

High energy
Stir in 10 mL (2 tsp) or more butter or margarine to hot cereal before adding sweetener.
Top with cream.

* Refer to Enriched Milk recipe.

GRANOLA

12-125 mL ($\frac{1}{2}$ cup) servings

Ingredients

750 mL	Rolled oats	3 cups
125 mL	Wheat germ	$\frac{1}{2}$ cup
125 mL	Shredded coconut	$\frac{1}{2}$ cup
50 mL	Bran	$\frac{1}{4}$ cup
50 mL	Sunflower seeds	$\frac{1}{4}$ cup
125 mL	Peanuts, chopped	$\frac{1}{2}$ cup
50 mL	Skim milk powder	$\frac{1}{4}$ cup
50 mL	Vegetable oil	$\frac{1}{4}$ cup
30 mL	Orange juice concentrate	2 tbsp
80 mL	Honey	$\frac{1}{3}$ cup
80 mL	Raisins	$\frac{1}{3}$ cup
50 mL	Apricots, dried, chopped	$\frac{1}{4}$ cup

Preheat oven to 180°C (350°F). Combine oats, wheat germ, coconut, bran, sunflower seeds, peanuts, and skim milk powder in large bowl. In separate bowl, combine vegetable oil, orange juice, and honey. Add wet ingredients to dry ingredients, mixing until dry ingredients are well coated. (Add more oil and honey if required.) Spread mixture evenly onto cookie sheet. Bake, stirring often to ensure even browning. (Mixture is done when light brown and crisp.) Remove from oven and stir in raisins and apricots. Cool and store in airtight jar.

Serving Suggestions

Serve at breakfast with milk or cream, topped with fresh fruit.

A great high-energy snack idea.

Nutrients per Serving

Energy	1134 kJ	Vitamin C	3 mg
	270 kcal	Calcium	47 mg
Protein	8.5 g	Potassium	305 mg
Fat	12 g	Iron	2 mg

Vitamin A	224 IU	Zinc	1 mg
Folacin	15 μg	Fiber	3.2 g
Vitamin B_{12}	0.1 μg		

Dietary Modifications

Restricted lactose
Omit skim milk powder.

Restrictions

This recipe is not suitable for a restricted-fat diet or restricted-fiber diet.

OVEN FRENCH TOAST

2 servings

Ingredients

3	Eggs		
180 mL	Enriched milk*	$\frac{3}{4}$ cup	
15 mL	Sugar	1 tbsp	
5 mL	Vanilla	1 tsp	
pinch	Salt		
4 slices	Whole-wheat bread, day-old		

Heat oven to 260°C (500°F). In a bowl, combine all ingredients except bread, beating until fluffy. Dip bread into egg mixture and arrange on greased baking sheet. Bake approximately 8 minutes on each side, or until golden brown.

Serving Suggestions

Serve hot.

A high-protein breakfast or brunch idea.

Top with one or more of the following:

    Butter and syrup
    Whipping cream
    Pureed peaches with a pinch of ginger
    Honey and butter heated and thinned with lemon juice
    Cooked frozen cranberries, blueberries, rhubarb, or strawberries
    Warmed apple or cherry pie filling
    Sliced fresh or canned fruit

Nutrients per Serving

Energy	1344 kJ	Vitamin C	1 mg
	320 kcal	Calcium	284 mg
Protein	18.6 g	Potassium	476 mg
Fat	10.9 g	Iron	2.2 mg
Vitamin A	520 IU	Zinc	2.2 mg
Folacin	63 μg	Fiber	3.0 g
Vitamin B$_{12}$	1.2 μg		

Dietary Modifications

Restricted lactose
Use milk-free bread if you are highly lactose intolerant.
Replace enriched milk with milk treated with a commercial lactase enzyme product.

Restricted fat
Replace enriched milk* with skim milk.
Reduce eggs to two.

Restricted fiber
Replace whole-wheat bread with white bread.

* Refer to Enriched Milk recipe.

FRUIT PANCAKES

5 servings (2 pancakes per serving)

Ingredients

1	Egg, beaten	
250 mL	2% milk	1 cup
30 mL	Vegetable oil	2 tbsp
250 mL	All-purpose flour	1 cup
30 mL	Brown sugar	2 tbsp
10 mL	Baking powder	2 tsp
1 mL	Salt	$\frac{1}{4}$ tsp
125 mL	Fresh fruit, cut-up	$\frac{1}{2}$ cup

Heat griddle or frying pan. In bowl, combine beaten egg, milk, and oil. In separate bowl, combine flour, sugar, baking powder, and salt. Combine wet and dry ingredients together, mixing gently until just combined (batter should be lumpy). Very gently fold in fruit. Pour batter onto lightly greased hot griddle (pancake should spread to about 10 cm (4 in) in diameter). Turn pancakes as they become puffy, full of bubbles, and slightly dry around the edges. Turn once only. Remove from heat once browned.

Serving Suggestions

Serve immediately.

Any fruit can be used—chopped apple, sliced banana, blueberries, strawberries, diced peaches, and so on.

Top with sliced fruit, plain or fruit yogurt, maple syrup, and so forth.

A nutritious breakfast, brunch, or lunch.

For a heartier meal, serve with bacon, ham, or sausages, and a glass of milk.

Nutrients per Serving

Energy	445 kJ	Vitamin C	2 mg
	106 kcal	Calcium	40 mg
Protein	2.8 g	Potassium	93 mg
Fat	3.8 g	Iron	0.8 mg

Vitamin A	90 IU	Zinc	0.3 mg
Folacin	8 µg	Fiber	0.7 g
Vitamin B$_{12}$	0.1 µg		

Dietary Modifications

Restricted lactose
   Use milk treated with a commercial lactase enzyme product.

Restricted fat
   Reduce oil to 15 mL (1 tbsp).
   Use skim milk in place of 2% milk.

Restricted fiber
   Choose fruit allowed on a restricted-fiber diet.

High protein
   Reduce milk by 30 mL (2 tbsp) and add an extra egg.
   Add 50 mL ($\frac{1}{4}$ cup) skim milk powder to dry ingredients.

High energy
   Replace 2% milk with whole milk.

CHEESE BISCUITS

12-5 cm (2 in) biscuits; 1 biscuit per serving

Ingredients

250 mL	All-purpose flour	1 cup
250 mL	Whole-wheat flour	1 cup
15 mL	Baking powder	1 tbsp
5 mL	Salt	1 tsp
80 mL	Margarine	$\frac{1}{3}$ cup
180 mL	2% milk	$\frac{3}{4}$ cup
125 mL	Cheddar cheese, shredded	$\frac{1}{2}$ cup

Heat oven to 230°C (450°F). Measure flour, baking powder, and salt into bowl. Cut in margarine thoroughly until mixture looks like crumbs the size of small peas. Stir in milk and cheese with fork until mixture leaves sides of bowl. Form dough into a ball, and, on a lightly floured surface, knead lightly about 10 times. Roll out dough to 1.25 cm ($\frac{1}{2}$ in) thick. Cut with a floured biscuit cutter or similar utensil. Arrange on ungreased baking sheet. Bake 10 to 15 minutes, or until lightly browned.

Serving Suggestions

Serve hot or cold with butter or jam.

Biscuits can be served at breakfast in place of toast, at lunch with soup and a salad, at supper with chili or stew, or as a between-meal snack.

Nutrients per Serving

Energy	630 kJ	Vitamin C	0 mg
	150 kcal	Calcium	108 mg
Protein	4.3 g	Potassium	44 mg
Fat	7.3 g	Iron	1 mg
Vitamin A	295 IU	Zinc	0.3 mg
Folacin	5 μg	Fiber	1.2 g
Vitamin B_{12}	0.1 μg		

Dietary Modifications

Restricted lactose
   Use milk treated with a commercial lactase enzyme product.
   Use milk-free margarine if you are highly lactose intolerant.

Restricted fat
   Use skim milk.
   Choose lower-fat cheese.
   Reduce margarine to 50 mL ($\frac{1}{4}$ cup).

Restricted fiber
   Replace whole-wheat flour with white flour.

High protein
   Add 50 mL ($\frac{1}{4}$ cup) skim milk powder to the dry ingredients.

High energy
   Follow high protein suggestion.
   Increase margarine to 125 mL ($\frac{1}{2}$ cup).

Restrictions

This recipe may be unsuitable for those with lactose intolerance if cheese is not well tolerated.

SCONES

12 servings

Ingredients

375 mL	All-purpose flour	$1\frac{1}{2}$ cups
125 mL	Brown sugar	$\frac{1}{2}$ cup
5 mL	Baking powder	1 tsp
1 mL	Salt	$\frac{1}{4}$ tsp
125 mL	Margarine	$\frac{1}{2}$ cup
125 mL	2% milk	$\frac{1}{2}$ cup
1	Egg, separated	
125 mL	Raisins	$\frac{1}{2}$ cup

Combine flour, sugar, baking powder, and salt in mixing bowl. Cut in margarine with pastry blender, until mixture looks like meal. Add milk, beaten egg white, and raisins, and combine gently. Form dough into ball and knead gently on floured surface about 8 times. Divide dough in half and roll each piece into a round until 1.25 cm ($\frac{1}{2}$ inch) thick. Beat egg yolk. Brush top of each round with egg yolk, and cut each into sixths. Place scones on ungreased baking sheet and bake at 230°C (450°F) 10 to 12 minutes, or until golden brown.

Serving Suggestions

Serve hot from the oven with butter, jam, or honey.

Can be served as a sweet bread for breakfast, a snack, or dessert.

Nutrients per Serving

Energy	777 kJ	Vitamin C	0 mg
	185 kcal	Calcium	45 mg
Protein	2.6 g	Potassium	110 mg
Fat	8.8 g	Iron	1.2 mg
Vitamin A	380 IU	Zinc	0.2 mg
Folacin	7 μg	Fiber	0.8 g
Vitamin B$_{12}$	0.1 μg		

Dietary Modifications

Restricted lactose
Use milk treated with a commercial lactase enzyme product.
Use milk-free margarine if you are highly lactose intolerant.

Restricted fat
Use skim milk in place of 2% milk.
Reduce margarine to 80 mL ($\frac{1}{3}$ cup).

Restricted fiber
Omit raisins.

High protein
Add 30 mL (2 tbsp) skim milk powder to dry ingredients.

High energy
Follow high protein suggestion.
Use whole milk in place of 2% milk.
Top with extra margarine or butter.

CORN BREAD

6 servings

Ingredients

250 mL	All-purpose flour	1 cup
180 mL	Cornmeal	$\frac{3}{4}$ cup
80 mL	Sugar	$\frac{1}{3}$ cup
10 mL	Baking powder	2 tsp
2 mL	Baking soda	$\frac{1}{2}$ tsp
2 mL	Salt	$\frac{1}{2}$ tsp
250 mL	Plain yogurt	1 cup
50 mL	Vegetable oil	$\frac{1}{4}$ cup
2	Eggs	

Preheat oven to 200°C (400°F). Grease 20 cm (8 in) square baking pan. In a bowl, stir together all dry ingredients. In a separate bowl, combine all wet ingredients, beating until smooth. Add wet ingredients to dry, folding together only until moistened. Pour batter into pan and bake approximately 25 minutes.

Serving Suggestions

Cut into squares, butter, and serve hot at lunch or supper with soup, chili, or stew. Butter, drizzle with maple syrup, and serve warm or cold at breakfast.

Nutrients per Serving

Energy	1260 kJ	Vitamin C	0 mg
	300 kcal	Calcium	137 mg
Protein	7 g	Potassium	124 mg
Fat	10.8 g	Iron	1.5 mg
Vitamin A	215 IU	Zinc	0.7 mg
Folacin	14 μg	Fiber	1.6 g
Vitamin B$_{12}$	0.3 μg		

Dietary Modifications

Restricted lactose
Choose yogurt that does not contain added milk solids.

Restricted fat
Use low-fat yogurt.
Reduce oil to 30 mL (2 tbsp).

High protein
Add 50 mL ($\frac{1}{4}$ cup) skim milk powder to dry ingredients.
Add 50 mL ($\frac{1}{4}$ cup) grated cheese to wet ingredients.

High energy
Follow high protein suggestions.
Increase oil to 80 mL ($\frac{1}{3}$ cup).
Use high-fat yogurt.

Restrictions

If one is highly lactose intolerant, this recipe may not be well tolerated.

DUMPLINGS

5 servings (2 dumplings per serving)

Ingredients

500 mL	All-purpose flour	2 cups
10 mL	Baking powder	2 tsp
5 mL	Salt	1 tsp
45 mL	Margarine	3 tbsp
200 mL	2% milk	$\frac{7}{8}$ cup

In a bowl, combine dry ingredients. Using a pastry blender or fork, cut margarine into dry ingredients until mixture forms crumbs the size of small peas. Stir in milk. Drop dough by tablespoons onto gently simmering soup or stew. Cook uncovered for 10 minutes. Cover and cook for 5 to 10 more minutes or until dumplings are fluffy.

Serving Suggestions

Serve hot with a hearty soup or stew.

Nutrients per Serving

Energy	1155 kJ	Vitamin C	0 mg
	275 kcal	Calcium	138 mg
Protein	6.9 g	Potassium	126 mg
Fat	8.2 g	Iron	2.5 mg
Vitamin A	368 IU	Zinc	0.5 mg
Folacin	16 μg	Fiber	1.4 g
Vitamin B$_{12}$	0.2 μg		

Dietary Modifications

Restricted lactose
   Use milk treated with a commercial lactase enzyme product.
   Use milk-free margarine if you are highly lactose intolerant.

Restricted fat
   Use skim milk in place of 2% milk.
   Reduce margarine to 30 mL (2 tbsp).

High protein
   Add 50 mL ($\frac{1}{4}$ cup) skim milk powder to dry ingredients.
   Add 50 mL ($\frac{1}{4}$ cup) grated cheese to flour mixture.

High energy
   Follow high protein suggestions.
   Replace 2% milk with whole milk.

FRIED RICE

4 servings

Ingredients

30 mL	Vegetable oil	2 tbsp
1	Green onion, chopped	
1	Garlic clove, minced	
1000 mL	Rice, cooked, cold	4 cups
pinch	Salt	
pinch	Pepper	

Heat oil in frying pan and sauté garlic and onion until tender. Add rice to pan and fry, stirring frequently, until rice is lightly browned. Add salt and pepper.

Serving Suggestions

Serve hot.

A tasty way to use up leftover rice.

Frying adds extra energy for those trying to gain weight.

Nutrients per Serving

Energy	1344 kJ	Vitamin C	1 mg
	320 kcal	Calcium	27 mg
Protein	6 g	Potassium	96 mg
Fat	7.5 g	Iron	2.4 mg
Vitamin A	1 IU	Zinc	1 mg
Folacin	9 μg	Fiber	1.2 g
Vitamin B$_{12}$	0 μg		

Dietary Modifications

Restricted fat
  Reduce oil to 15 mL (1 tbsp).

Restricted fiber
  Omit onion.

HONEY-NUT RICE

4 servings

Ingredients

15 mL	Margarine	1 tbsp
30 mL	Honey	2 tbsp
pinch	Cinnamon	
pinch	Salt	
750 mL	Rice, cooked, hot	3 cups
125 mL	Almonds, chopped	½ cup

Combine margarine, honey, cinnamon, and salt. Add to hot rice, combining well. Gently stir in nuts.

Serving Suggestions

Serve hot.

An excellent alternative to plain rice, served alone or at a meal with chicken, fish, or beef.

Nutrients per Serving

Energy	1470 kJ	Vitamin C	0 mg
	350 kcal	Calcium	65 mg
Protein	8 g	Potassium	196 mg
Fat	12.3 g	Iron	2.5 mg
Vitamin A	118 IU	Zinc	1.3 mg
Folacin	15 µg	Fiber	2.7 g
Vitamin B$_{12}$	0 µg		

Dietary Modifications

Restricted lactose
  Use milk-free margarine if you are highly lactose intolerant.

Restricted fat
  Reduce margarine to 10 mL (2 tsp).

Restricted fiber
  Omit nuts.

High energy
  Increase margarine to 30 mL (2 tbsp).

ORANGE-RAISIN RICE

4 servings

Ingredients

250 mL	Rice, regular, uncooked	1 cup
250 mL	Water, boiling	1 cup
250 mL	Orange juice, heated	1 cup
50 mL	Raisins	$\frac{1}{4}$ cup
2 mL	Salt	$\frac{1}{2}$ tsp
5 mL	Orange peel, grated	1 tsp

Preheat oven to 180°C (350°F). In a 1 L (1 qt) ungreased baking dish, combine all ingredients, mixing well. Cover tightly and bake for 25 to 30 minutes, or until rice is tender.

Serving Suggestions

Serve hot.

A tasty alternative to plain rice.

Serve with meat, fish, or poultry.

A handful of chopped peanuts will provide additional taste and texture.

Nutrients per Serving

Energy	520 kJ	Vitamin C	27 mg
	124 kcal	Calcium	26 mg
Protein	4 g	Potassium	228 mg
Fat	0.3 g	Iron	1.6 mg
Vitamin A	54 IU	Zinc	0.6 mg
Folacin	34 μg	Fiber	1 g
Vitamin B$_{12}$	0 μg		

Dietary Modifications

Restricted fiber
   Do not add raisins, peanuts, or orange peel.

High energy
   Stir 15 mL (1 tbsp) butter or margarine into rice before serving.

BARLEY BAKE

4 servings

Ingredients

15 mL	Margarine	1 tbsp
125 mL	Pot barley	$\frac{1}{2}$ cup
80 mL	Carrot, grated	$\frac{1}{3}$ cup
15 mL	Onion, finely chopped	1 tbsp
50 mL	Mushroom pieces, canned	$\frac{1}{4}$ cup
dash	Pepper	
5 mL	Beef bouillon powder	1 tsp
375 mL	Water, hot	$1\frac{1}{2}$ cups

Heat oven to 190°C (375°F). Melt margarine in frying pan. Add barley, carrot, and onion and cook until brown. Place in a 1 L (1 qt) baking dish. Add mushrooms and pepper. Dissolve bouillon powder in hot water and pour over ingredients in dish, stirring to mix. Cover and bake for approximately 45 minutes, or until barley is tender and liquid is absorbed.

Serving Suggestions

Serve hot as an accompaniment to meat, fish, or chicken.

An excellent alternative to potatoes, rice, or noodles.

A handful of nuts or seeds can be added for taste and texture variation.

Nutrients per Serving

Energy	525 kJ	Vitamin C	1 mg
	125 kcal	Calcium	14 mg
Protein	3 g	Potassium	133 mg
Fat	3.2 g	Iron	0.8 mg
Vitamin A	2734 IU	Zinc	0.8 mg
Folacin	8 μg	Fiber	4.9 g
Vitamin B$_{12}$	0 μg		

Dietary Modifications

Restricted lactose
   Use milk-free margarine if you are highly lactose intolerant.

Restricted fat
   Reduce margarine to 10 mL (2 tsp).

High energy
   Increase margarine to 30 mL (2 tbsp).

Restrictions

This recipe is unsuitable for a restricted-fiber diet.

10

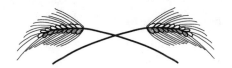

Vegetables

Oriental Vegetables
Herbed Green Beans
Marmalade Carrots
Carrots and Dill

Brussels Sprouts and
   Mushroom Bake
Creamed Cauliflower and Peas
Cheesy Potatoes
Stuffed Baked Potatoes

ORIENTAL VEGETABLES

4 servings

Ingredients

30 mL	Vegetable oil	2 tbsp
180 mL	Carrots, thinly sliced	$\frac{3}{4}$ cup
180 mL	Green beans, sliced	$\frac{3}{4}$ cup
180 mL	Cauliflowerets, thinly sliced	$\frac{3}{4}$ cup
125 mL	Green onions, sliced	$\frac{1}{2}$ cup
180 mL	Mushroom halves, fresh	$\frac{3}{4}$ cup
250 mL	Water	1 cup
10 mL	Chicken broth powder	2 tsp
10 mL	Cornstarch	2 tsp
pinch	Garlic powder	

Heat oil in a wok or frying pan until very hot. Stir-fry carrots and beans over medium heat for 1 to 2 minutes. Add cauliflower, onion, and mushroom and cook for 1 minute. Combine water, chicken broth powder, cornstarch, and garlic powder to make sauce. Add sauce to vegetables and stir until thickened; remove from heat.

Serving Suggestions

Serve hot.

An excellent cooking method for retaining the nutritional value of vegetables.

Replace one or more vegetables with an equal amount of asparagus, broccoli, zucchini, or celery.

Nutrients per Serving

Energy	395 kJ	Vitamin C	23 mg
	94 kcal	Calcium	26 mg
Protein	1.4 g	Potassium	242 mg
Fat	7.1 g	Iron	0.8 mg

Vitamin A	5725 IU	Zinc	0.3 mg
Folacin	25 μg	Fiber	1.4 g
Vitamin B_{12}	0 μg		

Dietary Modifications

Restricted fat
   Reduce oil to 15 mL (1 tbsp).

Restricted fiber
   Omit onions.
   If cauliflower is not well tolerated, replace with cubed eggplant.

HERBED GREEN BEANS

4 servings

Ingredients

500 mL	Green beans, fresh	2 cups
10 mL	Margarine, melted	2 tsp
10 mL	Lemon juice	2 tsp
pinch	Oregano	
5 mL	Pimiento, finely chopped	1 tsp
pinch	Salt	
pinch	Pepper	
pinch	Garlic powder	
30 mL	Croutons, crushed	2 tbsp

Cook green beans in boiling salted water until tender, about 10 to 15 minutes. Drain and toss with margarine. Mix together all other ingredients, except croutons. Pour over beans, toss, and arrange in a serving dish. Garnish with croutons.

Serving Suggestions

Serve hot.

An easy way to spice up a common vegetable.

Nutrients per Serving

Energy	273 kJ	Vitamin C	11 mg
	65 kcal	Calcium	27 mg
Protein	1.8 g	Potassium	137 mg
Fat	2.7 g	Iron	0.7 mg
Vitamin A	468 IU	Zinc	0.2 mg
Folacin	22 μg	Fiber	1.5 g
Vitamin B$_{12}$	0 μg		

Dietary Modifications

Restricted lactose
Use milk-free margarine if you are highly lactose intolerant.

Restricted fat
Reduce margarine to 5 mL (1 tsp).

High energy
Increase margarine to 15 mL (1 tbsp) or more.
Add more croutons.

Restrictions

This recipe is unsuitable for a restricted-fiber diet.

MARMALADE CARROTS

4 servings

Ingredients

500 mL	Carrots, raw, diced	2 cups
50 mL	Orange juice	$\frac{1}{4}$ cup
pinch	Salt	
30 mL	Orange marmalade	2 tbsp
15 mL	Margarine	1 tbsp
15 mL	Brown sugar	1 tbsp

Combine all ingredients except margarine and brown sugar. Place in 1 L (1 qt) casserole dish and lightly dot with margarine. Cover and bake in 180°C (350°F) oven for 20 to 25 minutes, or until carrots are tender. Sprinkle with brown sugar just before cooking is complete.

Serving Suggestions

Serve hot.

A sweet and tasty way to prepare a common vegetable.

Nutrients per Serving

Energy	407 kJ	Vitamin C	12 mg
	97 kcal	Calcium	27 mg
Protein	0.9 g	Potassium	272 mg
Fat	3 g	Iron	0.5 mg
Vitamin A	20,500 IU	Zinc	0.2 mg
Folacin	16 μg	Fiber	2.4 g
Vitamin B$_{12}$	0 μg		

Dietary Modifications

Resticted lactose
   Use milk-free margarine if you are highly lactose intolerant.

Restricted fat
   Reduce margarine to 10 mL (2 tsp).

Restricted fiber
   Omit marmalade and replace with jelly.

CARROTS AND DILL

4 servings

Ingredients

50 mL	Whole milk	$\frac{1}{4}$ cup	
125 mL	Mayonnaise	$\frac{1}{2}$ cup	
1–2 mL	Lemon juice	$\frac{1}{4}-\frac{1}{2}$ tsp	
pinch	Dill		
500 mL	Carrots, cooked	2 cups	

In a small saucepan, slowly combine milk with mayonnaise. Add lemon juice and dill. Stir over low heat for 1 to 2 minutes until thoroughly mixed and heated through. Remove from heat and pour over cooked carrots.

Serving Suggestions

Serve hot as an accompaniment to a roast beef or baked fish dinner.
An excellent way to dress up vegetables.
A tasty high-energy vegetable recipe.

Nutrients per Serving

Energy	1037 kJ	Vitamin C	7 mg
	247 kcal	Calcium	40 mg
Protein	1.5 g	Potassium	264 mg
Fat	23.6 g	Iron	0.5 mg
Vitamin A	20,450 IU	Zinc	0.2 mg
Folacin	11 μg	Fiber	2.3 g
Vitamin B_{12}	0.1 μg		

Dietary Modifications

Restricted lactose
Use milk treated with a commercial lactase enzyme product.
Use pure mayonnaise, not a mayonnaise substitute.

High protein
Add 30 mL (2 tbsp) skim milk powder to milk and mayonnaise mixture.

High energy
Follow high protein suggestion.

Restrictions

This recipe is not suitable for a restricted-fat diet.

BRUSSELS SPROUTS AND MUSHROOM BAKE

4 servings

Ingredients

15 mL	Butter or margarine	1 tbsp
500 mL	Brussels sprouts	2 cups
250 mL	Mushrooms, sliced	1 cup
$\frac{1}{2}$ small	Red pepper, diced	
dash	Salt	
dash	Pepper	
160 mL	Swiss cheese, grated	$\frac{2}{3}$ cup

Preheat oven to 180°C (350°F). Melt butter in frying pan and sauté vegetables lightly. Season with salt and pepper. Place in casserole dish. Top with grated cheese and bake for 20 to 25 minutes.

Serving Suggestions

Serve hot.

An excellent accompaniment to chicken and rice.

An easy way to improve calcium and protein intake.

Nutrients per Serving

Energy	609 kJ		Vitamin C	96 mg
	145 kcal		Calcium	235 mg
Protein	8.6 g		Potassium	362 mg
Fat	9.2 g		Iron	1.4 mg
Vitamin A	1500 IU		Zinc	1.2 mg
Folacin	56 μg		Fiber	1.6 g
Vitamin B$_{12}$	0.4 μg			

Dietary Modifications

Restricted lactose
 Use milk-free margarine if you are highly lactose intolerant.

Restricted fat
 Reduce butter to 5 mL (1 tsp).
 Replace Swiss cheese with low-fat mozzarella cheese.

Restrictions

Because of the cheese content, this recipe may be unsuitable for a restricted-lactose diet if one is significantly lactose intolerant. This recipe is unsuitable for a restricted-fiber diet.

CREAMED CAULIFLOWER AND PEAS

4 servings

Ingredients

15 mL	Margarine	1 tbsp
15 mL	All-purpose flour	1 tbsp
1 mL	Salt	$\frac{1}{4}$ tsp
dash	Pepper	
250 mL	2% milk	1 cup
250 mL	Peas, cooked	1 cup
250 mL	Cauliflower, cooked	1 cup
50 mL	Cheddar cheese, grated	$\frac{1}{4}$ cup

In a saucepan, melt margarine over low heat. Stir in flour, salt, and pepper until well blended. Remove from heat and stir in milk. Return to heat, stirring constantly just until boiling. Continue to cook for 1 minute. Add vegetables and stir just until heated through. Top with Cheddar cheese.

Serving Suggestions

Serve hot topped with grated cheese and parsley.

May be served over toast as a light meal.

An excellent way to use leftover vegetables.

A tasty, calcium-rich, high-energy, high-protein vegetable dish.

Nutrients per Serving

Energy	546 kJ	Vitamin C	34 mg
	130 kcal	Calcium	142 mg
Protein	6.5 g	Potassium	309 mg
Fat	6.3 g	Iron	0.9 mg
Vitamin A	565 IU	Zinc	1 mg
Folacin	47 μg	Fiber	2.1 g
Vitamin B$_{12}$	0.3 μg		

Dietary Modifications

Restricted fat
Use skim milk.

Restricted fiber
Replace peas with mushrooms.
If cauliflower is not well-tolerated, replace with carrots.

High protein
Add 50 mL ($\frac{1}{4}$ cup) skim milk powder to milk.
Top with extra cheese.

High energy
Follow high protein suggestions.
Use whole milk in place of 2% milk.

Restrictions

This recipe is not suitable for a restricted-lactose diet.

CHEESY POTATOES

6 servings

Ingredients

6 medium	Potatoes, peeled	
1 mL	Salt	$\frac{1}{4}$ tsp
1 mL	Pepper	$\frac{1}{4}$ tsp
2 mL	Garlic powder	$\frac{1}{2}$ tsp
1 mL	Nutmeg	$\frac{1}{4}$ tsp
30 mL	All-purpose flour	1 tbsp
180 mL	Whole milk	$\frac{3}{4}$ cup
250 mL	Swiss cheese, grated	1 cup

Slice potatoes very thinly and arrange one-third in the bottom of a greased 3 L (3 qt) baking dish. Combine salt, pepper, garlic powder, nutmeg, and flour. Sprinkle one-third of this mixture and one-third of cheese over the first layer. Repeat twice. Pour milk over top layer. Cover and bake for 1 hour at 180°C (350°F), or until potatoes are tender and cheese is golden brown and bubbly.

Serving Suggestions

Serve hot.

Garnish with parsley before serving.

An interesting alternative to scalloped potatoes.

Try using different types of cheese, or adding crumbled fried slices of bacon or cubes of ham.

Nutrients per Serving

Energy	1050 kJ	Vitamin C	20 mg
	250 kcal	Calcium	228 mg
Protein	9.7 g	Potassium	672 mg
Fat	6.4 g	Iron	0.7 mg
Vitamin A	200 IU	Zinc	1.3 mg
Folacin	17 μg	Fiber	1.2 g
Vitamin B_{12}	0.4 μg		

Dietary Modifications

Restricted lactose
   Use milk treated with a commercial lactase enzyme product.

Restricted fat
   Replace whole milk with skim milk.
   Replace Swiss cheese with low-fat cheese.

High protein
   Replace whole milk with enriched milk.*

Restrictions

Because of the cheese content, this recipe may not be well tolerated by individuals who are significantly lactose intolerant.

* Refer to Enriched Milk recipe.

STUFFED BAKED POTATOES

4 servings

Ingredients

4 large	Baking potatoes, scrubbed	
50 mL	2% milk	$\frac{1}{4}$ cup
50 mL	Margarine, melted	$\frac{1}{4}$ cup
dash	Salt	
dash	Pepper	
2 slices	Bacon, crisply fried, drained	
30 mL	Parsley, minced	2 tbsp

Rub potatoes lightly with oil for softer skins. Prick skins with fork to allow steam to escape. Bake in 190°C (375°F) oven for 1 to 1 1/4 hours, or until potatoes are done. Cut off tops of potatoes lengthwise and scoop out centers into bowl, keeping skin intact. Mash potato and stir in milk, one-half of margarine, salt, and pepper. Crumble in bacon, add parsley, and mix well. Pack potato mixture into potato-skin shells. Drizzle tops with remaining margarine. Return to oven and broil 12.5 cm (5 in) from heat. Remove from oven when tops are browned.

Serving Suggestions

Serve immediately.

An appetizing accompaniment to any main meal.

An appealing alternative to more traditionally prepared potatoes.

Nutrients per Serving

Energy	1323 kJ	Vitamin C	33 mg
	315 kcal	Calcium	42 mg
Protein	6.5 g	Potassium	945 mg
Fat	11 g	Iron	2.7 mg
Vitamin A	483 IU	Zinc	0.9 mg
Folacin	29 μg	Fiber	3.7 g
Vitamin B$_{12}$	0.1 μg		

Dietary Modifications

Restricted lactose

Use milk treated with a commercial lactase enzyme product.
Use milk-free margarine if you are highly lactose intolerant.

Restricted fat

Reduce margarine to 15 mL (1 tbsp).
Use skim milk.
Drain bacon well.

Restricted fiber

Do not eat potato skin.

High protein

Stir in 15 mL (1 tbsp) skim milk powder to potato mixture.
Add 80 mL ($\frac{1}{3}$ cup) grated cheese to potato mixture.

High energy

Follow high protein suggestions.
Use cream in place of milk.
Drizzle with extra margarine.

11

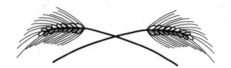

Entrées

Creamy High-Protein Omelet

Crustless Quiche

Frittata

Three-Cheese Vegetable Casserole

Fabulous Fettuccine

Citrus Chicken

Baked Salmon Squares

Clam Casserole

Almond Pork

One-Dish Delight

Chili

Asparagus Sukiyaki

Easy Curried Beef

Beef and Vegetable Stir Fry

CREAMY HIGH-PROTEIN OMELET

2 servings

Ingredients

2	Eggs, lightly beaten	
250 mL	2% cottage cheese	1 cup
125 mL	Cheddar cheese, mild, grated	$\frac{1}{2}$ cup
pinch	Dill	

Preheat oven to 230°C (450°F). Grease a medium-sized oven dish. In a bowl, combine beaten eggs with cottage cheese, mixing lightly. Pour mixture into oven dish and sprinkle with Cheddar cheese and dill. Bake for 10 minutes.

Serving Suggestions

Cut in half and serve immediately.

Serve with hot buttered toast, bagels, or muffins.

An excellent breakfast or light lunch idea.

A light, high-energy, high-protein meal on days when appetite is poor.

Nutrients per Serving

Energy	1113 kJ	Vitamin C	0 mg
	265 kcal	Calcium	293 mg
Protein	24.3 g	Potassium	160 mg
Fat	16.5 g	Iron	1.2 mg
Vitamin A	690 IU	Zinc	1.83 mg
Folacin	38 μg	Fiber	0 g
Vitamin B$_{12}$	1.24 μg		

Restrictions

This recipe is not suitable for a restricted-lactose diet or restricted-fat diet.

CRUSTLESS QUICHE

4 servings

Ingredients

15 mL	Butter or margarine	1 tbsp
125 mL	Onion, sliced	$\frac{1}{2}$ cup
125 mL	Mushrooms, fresh, sliced	$\frac{1}{2}$ cup
125 mL	Ham, cooked, diced	$\frac{1}{2}$ cup
4	Eggs	
125 mL	Whole milk	$\frac{1}{2}$ cup
3 mL	Salt	$\frac{3}{4}$ tsp
pinch	Pepper	
50 mL	Swiss cheese, grated	$\frac{1}{4}$ cup

In a frying pan, melt butter. Add onions and mushrooms and sauté until they are limp. Spread mixture into bottom of greased 22.5 cm (9 in) pie plate and top with ham. Beat together eggs, milk, salt, and pepper. Pour mixture over onions, mushrooms, and ham. Sprinkle with cheese. Bake for 30 to 40 minutes at 180°C (350°F), or until knife inserted in center comes out clean.

Serving Suggestions

Let stand for 5 minutes to set; then slice and serve.

An excellent brunch dish.

Ham can be replaced with an equal amount of chicken, pork, or beef.

Nutrients per Serving

Energy	798 kJ	Vitamin C	2 mg
	190 kcal	Calcium	138 mg
Protein	14 g	Potassium	254 mg
Fat	12.7 g	Iron	1.2 mg
Vitamin A	435 IU	Zinc	1.8 mg
Folacin	30 μg	Fiber	0.3 g
Vitamin B_{12}	0.9 μg		

Dietary Modifications

Restricted lactose
Use milk treated with a commercial lactase enzyme product.
Use milk-free margarine if you are highly lactose intolerant.

Restricted fiber
Omit onions.

Restricted fat
Reduce butter to 5 mL (1 tsp).
Replace whole milk with skim milk.
Replace Swiss cheese with a lower-fat cheese.

High protein
Replace whole milk with enriched milk.*
Increase cheese to 125 mL ($\frac{1}{2}$ cup).

Restrictions

If you are highly lactose intolerant, this recipe may not be well tolerated because of the cheese content.

* See Enriched Milk recipe

FRITTATA

4 servings

Ingredients

80 mL	Onion, finely chopped	$\frac{1}{3}$ cup
80 mL	Green pepper, chopped	$\frac{1}{3}$ cup
20 mL	Margarine	4 tsp
8 medium	Eggs, beaten	
125 mL	2% milk	$\frac{1}{2}$ cup
5 mL	Salt	1 tsp
5 mL	Worcestershire sauce	1 tsp
450 mL	Rice, cooked	$1\frac{3}{4}$ cups
1 medium	Tomato, chopped	
125 mL	Cheddar cheese, shredded	$\frac{1}{2}$ cup

Sauté onions and pepper in margarine until tender. In a bowl, combine beaten eggs with milk, salt, and Worcestershire sauce. Add onions, pepper, rice, and tomato to egg mixture. Pour into a medium-sized flat-bottomed frying pan or skillet. Cover and cook over medium-low heat for 15 minutes or until top is set. Evenly cover top with grated cheese. Remove from heat, cover, and let sit for 5 minutes to allow egg to set and cheese to melt.

Serving Suggestions

Quarter and serve hot.

An excellent brunch idea.

Serve with biscuits, a salad, and a glass of milk for a complete meal.

A delicious high-energy, high-protein meal.

Nutrients per Serving

Energy	1596 kJ	Vitamin C	23 mg
	380 kcal	Calcium	206 mg
Protein	18.7 g	Potassium	324 mg
Fat	18.5 g	Iron	2.8 mg
Vitamin A	1187 IU	Zinc	2 mg
Folacin	57 μg	Fiber	1.3 g
Vitamin B$_{12}$	1.1 μg		

Dietary Modifications

Restricted lactose
   Use milk treated with a commercial lactase enzyme product.
   Use milk-free margarine if you are highly lactose intolerant.

Restricted fiber
   Remove skin and seeds from tomato.
   Omit green pepper and onion and replace with 125 mL ($\frac{1}{2}$ cup) sliced
   mushrooms.

High protein
   Add 30 mL (2 tbsp) skim milk powder to egg and milk mixture.
   Add extra cheese.

High energy
   Follow high protein suggestions.
   Increase margarine to 30 mL (2 tbsp).
   Use whole milk.

Restrictions

This recipe in not suitable for a restricted-fat diet. If you are highly lactose intolerant, this recipe may not be well tolerated because of the cheese content.

THREE-CHEESE VEGETABLE CASSEROLE

4 servings

Ingredients

1 kg	Zucchini, unpared, cut into 1.25 cm ($\frac{1}{2}$ in) slices	2 lb
500 mL	2% cottage cheese	2 cups
2 medium	Eggs, beaten	
300 mL	Rice, cooked	$1\frac{1}{4}$ cups
1 medium	Onion, finely diced	
30 mL	Chives, chopped	2 tbsp
dash	Pepper	
dash	Salt	
30 mL	Parmesan cheese, grated	2 tbsp
50 mL	Cheddar cheese, mild, grated	$\frac{1}{4}$ cup

Heat oven to 180°C (350°F). Lightly grease 1.5 L ($1\frac{1}{2}$ qt) casserole dish. In saucepan, bring 2.5 cm (1 in) of water to boiling. Add zucchini to water, cover, and return to boiling. Reduce heat and allow zucchini to cook for 10 to 15 minutes, or until tender. Remove from heat and drain. In a bowl, combine cottage cheese, egg, rice, onion, and spices. Arrange one-half of the zucchini in the casserole dish. Top with one-half of the cottage cheese and rice mixture. Repeat layers. Top with Parmesan and Cheddar cheese. Bake for 45 minutes, or until cheese is golden brown and bubbly.

Serving Suggestions

Serve hot.

A delicious, cheesy, high-protein, high-calcium dish.

A tasty alternative to a meat entrée.

Nutrients per Serving

Energy	1260 kJ	Vitamin C	26 mg
	300 kcal	Calcium	225 mg
Protein	27 g	Potassium	854 mg

Fat	8 g	Iron	2.4 mg
Vitamin A	1250 IU	Zinc	1.9 mg
Folacin	91 μg	Fiber	2.2 g
Vitamin B$_{12}$	1.1 μg		

Dietary Modifications

Restricted fat
   Use a lower-fat mild cheese.

Restricted fiber
   Pare zucchini and remove seeds.
   Omit onion and replace with 125 mL ($\frac{1}{2}$ cup) finely sliced mushrooms.

Restrictions

This recipe is unsuitable for a restricted-lactose diet.

FABULOUS FETTUCCINE

4 servings

Ingredients

225 g	Fettuccine, green, uncooked	$\frac{1}{2}$ lb
30 mL	Margarine	2 tbsp
80 mL	Mushrooms, fresh, sliced	$\frac{1}{3}$ cup
160 mL	Heavy cream	$\frac{2}{3}$ cup
125 mL	Red pepper, diced	$\frac{1}{2}$ cup
60 g	Ham, sliced into fine strips	2 oz
125 mL	Parmesan cheese, grated	$\frac{1}{2}$ cup
dash	Salt	
dash	Pepper	

Prepare fettuccine according to package directions; drain and set aside. In a frying pan, heat margarine. Add mushrooms and sauté until lightly browned. Add cream and boil for $1\frac{1}{2}$ minutes. Add red pepper. Reduce heat to low and stir in ham, cheese, and noodles. Gently toss mixture until well combined. Sprinkle with salt and pepper to taste.

Serving Suggestions

Serve immediately with a crisp salad and chunks of buttered French bread.

Nutrients per Serving

Energy	1995 kJ	Vitamin C	41 mg
	475 kcal	Calcium	187 mg
Protein	15 g	Potassium	248 mg
Fat	25 g	Iron	2.7 mg
Vitamin A	2031 IU	Zinc	1.5 mg
Folacin	18 μg	Fiber	1.8 g
Vitamin B$_{12}$	0.2 μg		

Dietary Modications

Restricted fiber

Omit red peppers, if not tolerated, and replace with extra mushrooms.

Restrictions

This recipe is not suitable for a restricted-lactose diet or a restricted-fat diet.

CITRUS CHICKEN

4 servings

Ingredients

2 large	Chicken breasts, halved	
45 mL	All-purpose flour	3 tbsp
5 mL	Paprika	1 tsp
5 mL	Salt	1 tsp
dash	Pepper	
30 mL	Butter or margarine	2 tbsp
15 mL	Orange rind, grated	1 tbsp
250 mL	Orange juice	1 cup
250 mL	Pineapple, crushed, undrained	1 cup
1 large	Orange, sliced	
6	Maraschino cherries	

Skin chicken and coat with mixture of flour, paprika, salt, and pepper. Sauté in butter or margarine until golden brown. Transfer to large casserole dish. Sprinkle with orange rind. Cover chicken with orange juice and pineapple. Cover and bake in preheated oven at 180°C (350°F) for one hour or until chicken is tender. Just before serving, place orange slices and cherries between chicken pieces and cook uncovered for 5 more minutes.

Serving Suggestions

Serve hot over plain rice or noodles.

An attractive, tasty dish.

Nutrients per Serving

Energy	1155 kJ	Vitamin C	52 mg
	275 kcal	Calcium	48 mg
Protein	28 g	Potassium	500 mg
Fat	9 g	Iron	1.5 mg
Vitamin A	750 IU	Zinc	1.1 mg
Folacin	43 μg	Fiber	1.5 g
Vitamin B$_{12}$	0.3 μg		

Dietary Modifications

Restricted lactose
Use milk-free margarine if you are highly lactose intolerant.

Restricted fat
Reduce butter to 15 mL (1 tbsp) or less.

Restricted fiber
Do not eat cherry or pineapple.
Do not add grated orange rind.

High energy
Do not remove skin from chicken.

BAKED SALMON SQUARES

4 servings

Ingredients

450 g	Salmon, canned, flaked, with bones	$15\frac{1}{2}$ oz
125 mL	Bread crumbs, dry	$\frac{1}{2}$ cup
2	Eggs, beaten	
1 can (300 g)	Cream of celery soup	$10\frac{3}{4}$ oz
50 mL	Sour cream	$\frac{1}{4}$ cup
50 mL	Onion, chopped	$\frac{1}{4}$ cup
pinch	Pepper	
pinch	Dill	

Combine all ingredients. Place in a 20 cm (8 in) lightly greased square baking dish. Bake uncovered at 160°C (325°F) for 1 hour or until brown on the sides and firm in the middle.

Serving Suggestions

Cut into squares before serving.
Serve with hot rolls, a salad, and a glass of milk for a nutritious, light meal.

Nutrients per Serving

Energy	1344 kJ	Vitamin C	1 mg
	320 kcal	Calcium	177 mg
Protein	21 g	Potassium	475 mg
Fat	16.5 g	Iron	2 mg
Vitamin A	437 IU	Zinc	1.1 mg
Folacin	34 μg	Fiber	0.9 g
Vitamin B_{12}	0.3 μg		

Dietary Modifications

Restricted fiber
    Omit onion.

Restrictions

This recipe is not suitable for a restricted-lactose diet or restricted-fat diet.

CLAM CASSEROLE

2 servings

Ingredients

125 mL	Baby clams, whole, canned	$\frac{1}{2}$ cup
250 mL	Brown rice, cooked	1 cup
30 mL	Green pepper, chopped	2 tbsp
50 mL	Onion, chopped	$\frac{1}{4}$ cup
1 large	Tomato, fresh, peeled, cubed	
dash	Salt	
dash	Pepper	
dash	Thyme	
80 mL	Cheddar cheese, mild, grated	$\frac{1}{3}$ cup

Preheat oven to 180°C (350°F). Combine all ingredients except cheese in a small baking dish. Top with cheese. Bake for 30 minutes or until heated through.

Serving Suggestions

Serve hot.

A quick meal for two.

Use wild or white rice in place of brown rice for variation.

Nutrients per Serving

Energy	1176 kJ	Vitamin C	29 mg
	280 kcal	Calcium	199 mg
Protein	19 g	Potassium	574 mg
Fat	8 g	Iron	13 mg
Vitamin A	1452 IU	Zinc	2.4 mg
Folacin	21 μg	Fiber	2.6 g
Vitamin B$_{12}$	42 μg		

Dietary Modifications

Restricted fiber
   Use white rice in place of brown rice.
   Omit onion.
   Omit green pepper, if not tolerated.
   Remove seeds from tomato.

Restrictions

Because of the cheese content, this recipe may be unsuitable for individuals who are significantly lactose intolerant.

ALMOND PORK

4 servings

Ingredients

30 mL	Margarine	2 tbsp
500 mL	Chicken bouillon	2 cups
30 mL	Cornstarch	2 tbsp
250 mL	Pineapple, crushed, undrained	1 cup
500 mL	Pork, cooked, cubed	2 cups
80 mL	Almonds, chopped	$\frac{1}{3}$ cup
80 mL	Green pepper, sliced	$\frac{1}{3}$ cup
2 mL	Salt	$\frac{1}{2}$ tsp

In a frying pan, melt margarine. Add chicken bouillon, bring to a boil, and reduce heat. In a small bowl, combine cornstarch and pineapple. Add pineapple mixture to bouillon, stirring frequently until mixture boils and thickens. Add pork, almonds, pepper, and salt. Allow mixture to come to a boil. Reduce heat and simmer for 8 to 10 minutes, or until heated through.

Serving Suggestions

Serve immediately over a bed of fluffy white rice.

An attractive tasty dish.

Chicken can be used in place of pork.

Nutrients per Serving

Energy	1365 kJ	Vitamin C	15 mg
	325 kcal	Calcium	52 mg
Protein	24 g	Potassium	357 mg
Fat	17 g	Iron	1.6 mg
Vitamin A	337 IU	Zinc	1.9 mg
Folacin	12 μg	Fiber	1.9 g
Vitamin B$_{12}$	0.3 μg		

Dietary Modifications

Restricted lactose
Use milk-free margarine of you are highly lactose intolerant.

Restricted Fat
Reduce margarine to 15 mL (1 tbsp).
Choose lean pork and trim all visible fat.

Restrictions

This recipe is not suitable for a restricted-fiber diet.

ONE-DISH DELIGHT

6 servings

Ingredients

4 slices	Bacon, chopped	
80 mL	Onion, chopped	$\frac{1}{3}$ cup
1 clove	Garlic, crushed	
1 medium	Red pepper, cut in strips	
1 medium	Green pepper, cut in strips	
80 mL	Mushrooms, fresh, sliced	$\frac{1}{3}$ cup
250 mL	Rice, uncooked	1 cup
1 can (796 mL)	Tomatoes, drained, chopped	28 oz
2 mL	Salt	$\frac{1}{2}$ tsp
pinch	Pepper	
pinch	Basil	
pinch	Oregano	
375 mL	Chicken broth	$1\frac{1}{2}$ cups
300 mL	Ham, cooked, cubed	$1\frac{1}{4}$ cups
15 medium	Shrimp, fresh, shelled	

Preheat oven to 180°C (350°F). Place greased shallow casserole dish in oven, allowing it to heat briefly. In a deep frying pan, fry bacon until crisp; remove and pat dry. Sauté onion and garlic in bacon fat over medium heat until lightly browned. Add peppers and mushrooms and continue to cook until just tender. Add rice, stirring frequently; cook until slightly opaque. Add tomatoes and spices, stirring to combine. Add bacon and broth and bring to boil. Stir in ham. Pour mixture into heated casserole dish. Cover and bake for 10 minutes. Push shrimp into mixture. Continue to cook for 15 to 20 minutes. Remove from oven when rice is tender and most of broth has been absorbed.

Serving Suggestions

Serve hot, garnished with sprigs of parsley.

An attractive dish to serve to guests.

Nutrients per Serving

Energy	1344 kJ	Vitamin C	59 mg
	320 kcal	Calcium	72 mg
Protein	20 g	Potassium	655 mg
Fat	10 g	Iron	4.1 mg
Vitamin A	1475 IU	Zinc	2.2 mg
Folacin	14 μg	Fiber	1.5 g
Vitamin B$_{12}$	0.8 μg		

Dietary Modifications

Restricted fat
Reduce bacon to two slices.

Restricted fiber
Remove seeds from tomatoes.
Omit onion.
Omit green and red peppers if not well tolerated. Replace with extra mushrooms or thin strips of carrot.

CHILI

4 large servings

Ingredients

450 g	Ground beef, lean	1 lb
250 mL	Onion, chopped	1 cup
1 medium	Green pepper, sliced	
500 mL	Red kidney beans, canned, undrained	2 cups
500 mL	Tomatoes, canned, undrained	2 cups
125 mL	Mushrooms, fresh, sliced	$\frac{1}{2}$ cup
250 mL	Tomato sauce	1 cup
15 mL	Garlic, minced	1 tbsp
7 mL	Mustard, prepared	$1\frac{1}{2}$ tsp
10 mL	Chili powder	2 tsp
5 mL	Salt	1 tsp
dash	Worcestershire sauce	
dash	Tobasco sauce	

Brown beef in deep frying pan. Drain excess fat. Add remaining ingredients and cook uncovered over low heat for 1 hour, stirring occasionally.

Serving Suggestions

Serve with a tossed salad and buttered whole-wheat rolls for a nutritious, iron-rich, high-fiber meal.

Nutrients per Serving

Energy	2050 kJ	Vitamin C	68 mg
	488 kcal	Calcium	123 mg
Protein	30 g	Potassium	1324 mg
Fat	15 g	Iron	5.6 mg
Vitamin A	1800 IU	Zinc	5.4 mg
Folacin	96 μg	Fiber	9 g
Vitamin B$_{12}$	2.6 μg		

Dietary Modifications

Restricted fat
Use very lean ground beef.
Remove as much fat as possible.

High protein
Top with grated Cheddar cheese before serving.

High energy
Follow high protein suggestion.
Use regular ground beef and do not drain off all the fat.

Restrictions

This recipe is unsuitable for a restricted-fiber diet.

ASPARAGUS SUKIYAKI

4 servings

Ingredients

250 g	Round steak	$\frac{1}{2}$ lb
1 clove	Garlic, mashed	
30 mL	Vegetable oil	2 tbsp
10 mL	Soy sauce	2 tsp
pinch	Salt	
30 mL	Water	2 tbsp
1 medium	Red pepper, cut in strips	
1 small	Onion, chopped	
500 g	Asparagus, fresh, cut into 5 cm (2 in) diagonal pieces	1 lb

In a frying pan or wok, heat oil until hot. Cut beef into thin diagonal strips. Brown beef and garlic in oil. Add soy sauce, salt, and water. Reduce heat; simmer uncovered for 8 to 10 minutes. Add vegetables and continue to cook for 5 to 8 minutes, or until asparagus is just tender.

Serving Suggestions

Serve immediately over plain rice or rice noodles.

Serve with extra soy sauce on the side.

A quick and easy nutritious meal.

Nutrients per Serving

Energy	1210 kJ	Vitamin C	79 mg
	288 kcal	Calcium	42 mg
Protein	15.5 g	Potassium	651 mg
Fat	22 g	Iron	2.4 mg

Vitamin A	2176 IU	Zinc	3 mg
Folacin	163 μg	Fiber	2.1 g
Vitamin B$_{12}$	1.7 μg		

Dietary Modifications

Restricted fat
Reduce oil to 15 mL (1 tbsp).
Remove all visible fat from meat.

Restrictions

This recipe is not suitable for a restricted-fiber diet.

EASY CURRIED BEEF

4 servings

Ingredients

1 can (300 mL)	Cream of mushroom soup	$10\frac{3}{4}$ oz
300 mL	2% milk	$1\frac{1}{4}$ cups
10 mL	Curry powder	2 tsp
pinch	Salt	
pinch	Pepper	
500 mL	Beef, cooked, cubed	2 cups

Combine soup, milk, and spices in saucepan. Add cubed beef. Cover and simmer for 25 to 30 minutes, or until meat is tender.

Serving Suggestions

Serve over a bed of steaming rice.

An easy and quick way to use leftover beef.

Serve with a crisp salad and a glass of milk for a complete meal.

Nutrients per Serving

Energy	1260 kJ	Vitamin C	1 mg
	300 kcal	Calcium	140 mg
Protein	20 g	Potassium	500 mg
Fat	13 g	Iron	2.3 mg
Vitamin A	169 IU	Zinc	5.6 mg
Folacin	10 μg	Fiber	0.6 g
Vitamin B_{12}	2.7 μg		

Dietary Modifications

Restricted fat
   Use skim milk.
   Use lean beef and trim all visible fat.

High protein
    Add extra meat.
    Add 50 mL ($\frac{1}{4}$ cup) skim milk powder to milk.

High energy
    Follow high protein suggestions.
    Use whole milk.

Restrictions

This recipe is not suitable for a restricted-lactose diet.

BEEF AND VEGETABLE STIR FRY

4 servings

Ingredients

125 mL	Beef broth	$\frac{1}{2}$ cup
30 mL	Soy sauce	2 tbsp
15 mL	Cornstarch	1 tbsp
5 mL	Sugar	1 tsp
450 g	Round steak, lean	1 lb
50 mL	Vegetable oil	$\frac{1}{4}$ cup
1 clove	Garlic, minced	
1	Onion, sliced in rings	
1 large	Carrot, thinly sliced	
1 medium	Red pepper, thinly sliced	
125 mL	Mushrooms, fresh, sliced	$\frac{1}{2}$ cup
250 mL	Snow peas	1 cup
750 mL	Rice, cooked	3 cups

In a small bowl, combine beef broth, soy sauce, cornstarch, and sugar. Set aside. Prepare beef by slicing into very thin diagonal strips. Heat wok or frying pan over high heat; then add 45 mL (3 tbsp) oil. Add garlic and beef and stir-fry until beef is lightly browned. Remove beef from wok and set aside. Heat remaining oil and stir-fry onions, carrots, pepper, and mushrooms until cooked but crisp. Add snowpeas and stir-fry briefly. Return meat to wok, add broth mixture, and stir until liquid thickens. Remove from heat. Serve over hot cooked rice.

Serving Suggestions

Beef can be replaced with chicken or pork.

Other vegetables such as cauliflower or zucchini can be used in place of vegetables listed.

Nutrients per Serving

Energy	2100 kJ	Vitamin C	72 mg
	500 kcal	Calcium	50 mg
Protein	28 g	Potassium	680 mg

Fat	21 g	Iron	5 mg
Vitamin A	6300 IU	Zinc	4.9 mg
Folacin	30 μg	Fiber	1.4 g
Vitamin B$_{12}$	2.5 μg		

Dietary Modifications

Restricted fat

Reduce oil to 5 to 10 mL (1 to 2 tsp).

Restricted fiber

Omit snowpeas and onion. Double amount of carrots and mushrooms. Omit green pepper if not well tolerated.

12

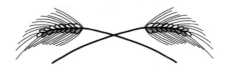

Desserts

FRUIT YOGURT

4 servings

Ingredients

500 mL	Plain yogurt	2 cups
160 mL	Strawberries, fresh, sliced	⅔ cup
1 medium	Banana, sliced	
50 mL	Almonds, chopped	¼ cup
30 mL	Maple syrup	2 tbsp
dash	Vanilla	

Gently combine all ingredients and spoon into 4 open-mouthed wine glasses.

Serving Suggestions

Serve chilled.

An excellent light dessert or snack.

Blueberries, peaches, or any other fruit can be used in place of strawberries.

Nutrients per Serving

Energy	756 kJ		Vitamin C	26 mg
	180 kcal		Calcium	180 mg
Protein	6.1 g		Potassium	435 mg
Fat	7.8 g		Iron	0.7 mg
Vitamin A	180 IU		Zinc	0.1 mg
Folacin	25 μg		Fiber	3 g
Vitamin B_{12}	0.5 μg			

Dietary Modifications

Restricted lactose
  Choose yogurt that does not contain added milk solids.

Restricted fat
Use low-fat yogurt.
Replace almonds with raisins.

Restricted fiber
Replace strawberries with peaches.
Omit nuts.

Restrictions

This recipe may be unsuitable for individuals who are significantly lactose intolerant.

EASY FRUIT SMOOTHIE

4 servings

Ingredients

1 pkg (30 g)	Vanilla instant pudding	1 oz
1 can (540 mL)	Fruit cocktail, packed in juice	19 oz
250 mL	Plain yogurt	1 cup
4	Maraschino cherries	

In a bowl, combine pudding mix with undrained fruit cocktail. Add yogurt and blend well. Spoon mixture into four dessert cups. Top each with a cherry and chill.

Serving Suggestions

Serve chilled as a light dessert or snack.

A quick and easy high-energy, high-protein dessert.

Nutrients per Serving

Energy	1105 kJ	Vitamin C	5 mg
	263 kcal	Calcium	278 mg
Protein	9.4 g	Potassium	348 mg
Fat	5.4 g	Iron	0.5 mg
Vitamin A	590 IU	Zinc	0.6 mg
Folacin	7 μg	Fiber	1 g
Vitamin B$_{12}$	0.4 μg		

Dietary Modifications

Restricted fat
    Choose low-fat yogurt.

Restricted fiber
    Remove fruit that contains skins.

High protein
    Add 50 mL ($\frac{1}{4}$ cup) skim milk powder to pudding mix.

High energy
    Use fruit cocktail packed in syrup.
    Use high-fat yogurt.

Restrictions

This recipe is unsuitable for a restricted-lactose diet.

COOKIE-TOPPED FRUITY PUDDING

6 servings

Ingredients

500 mL	Fruit, sliced, fresh or canned	2 cups
125 mL	Cookie crumbs	$\frac{1}{2}$ cup
80 mL	Sugar	$\frac{1}{3}$ cup
30 mL	Cornstarch	2 tbsp
pinch	Salt	
500 mL	2% milk	2 cups
2	Egg yolks, slightly beaten	
30 mL	Butter	2 tbsp
10 mL	Vanilla	2 tsp

Place 50 mL ($\frac{1}{4}$ cup) sliced mixed fruit into the bottom of four clear dessert dishes or wine glasses. Cover with 15 mL (1 tbsp) cookie crumbs. In a saucepan, combine sugar, cornstarch, and salt. Mix together milk and egg, and slowly add to sugar mixture. Stirring constantly, cook mixture over medium heat until thickened. Bring mixture to boil and continue to cook and stir for one minute. Remove from heat and stir in butter and vanilla. Allow to cool slightly. Spoon pudding into dessert glasses, covering cookie crumbs. Top pudding with remaining fruit and cookie crumbs. Chill.

Serving Suggestions

A high-energy, high-protein, nutritious dessert or snack idea.

Various fruits and fruit combinations can be used as well as various favorite cookie crumbs.

Nutrients per Serving

Energy	1134 kJ	Vitamin C	13 mg
	270 kcal	Calcium	130 mg
Protein	5.2 g	Potassium	329 mg
Fat	10.7 g	Iron	0.6 mg
Vitamin A	626 IU	Zinc	0.7 mg
Folacin	25 μg	Fiber	2 g
Vitamin B$_{12}$	0.5 μg		

Dietary Modifications

Restricted lactose
Choose cookies allowed on a restricted-lactose diet.
Use milk treated with a commercial lactase enzyme product.
Use milk-free margarine if you are highly lactose intolerant.

Restricted fat
Use skim milk.

Restricted fiber
Choose fruit allowed on a restricted-fiber diet.

High protein
Add 80 mL ($\frac{1}{3}$ cup) skim milk powder to milk.

High energy
Use whole milk in place of 2% milk.

RICE PUDDING

4 servings

Ingredients

250 mL	Whole milk	1 cup
3	Eggs	
5 mL	Vanilla	1 tsp
125 mL	Sugar	$\frac{1}{2}$ cup
2 mL	Lemon juice	$\frac{1}{2}$ tsp
500 mL	Rice, cooked, cooled	2 cups
80 mL	Raisins	$\frac{1}{3}$ cup
125 mL	Heavy cream	$\frac{1}{2}$ cup

Preheat oven to 180°C (350°F). In a blender, combine milk, eggs, vanilla, sugar, and lemon. Add rice and raisins and spread into greased 20 cm (8 in) square pan and bake, stirring mixture every 8 to 10 minutes. Remove from oven after 25 minutes. Cool for 10 minutes; then stir in heavy cream.

Serving Suggestions

Serve hot or cold as a dessert or snack.

Top with your favorite fruit or preserves for additional texture and flavor.

Nutrients per Serving

Energy	1890 kJ	Vitamin C	1 mg
	450 kcal	Calcium	128 mg
Protein	9 g	Potassium	285 mg
Fat	17.5 g	Iron	1.8 mg
Vitamin A	712 IU	Zinc	1.2 mg
Folacin	24 μg	Fiber	0.9 g
Vitamin B$_{12}$	0.7 μg		

Dietary Modifications

Restricted lactose

   Use milk treated with a commercial lactase enzyme product.
   Replace heavy cream with plain yogurt (no added milk solids).

Restricted fat
    Use skim milk in place of whole milk.
    Reduce eggs to two.
    Replace heavy cream with low-fat yogurt.

Restricted fiber
    Omit raisins and replace with 180 mL ($\frac{3}{4}$ cup) sliced peaches.

High protein
    Replace whole milk with enriched milk.*

Restrictions

This recipe is not suitable for a restricted-lactose diet if yogurt is not well tolerated.

* See Enriched Milk recipe.

APRICOT-RAISIN BREAD PUDDING

6 servings

Ingredients

1000 mL	Raisin bread, cubed	4 cups
500 mL	Whole milk	2 cups
30 mL	Margarine, melted	2 tbsp
3 medium	Eggs, slightly beaten	
80 mL	Sugar	$\frac{1}{3}$ cup
5 mL	Vanilla	1 tsp
80 mL	Apricots, dried, finely chopped	$\frac{1}{3}$ cup

Preheat oven to 180°C (350°F). Lightly grease 20 cm (8 in) square baking dish. Place bread in large bowl. Pour milk over bread and let stand for 15 minutes. Beat together margarine, eggs, sugar, and vanilla. Add egg mixture to bread, and stir until blended. Add chopped apricots. Pour into prepared pan. Bake for 30 to 40 minutes or until golden brown and knife inserted into center comes out clean.

Serving Suggestions

Serve hot or cold.

May be served alone or topped with whipped topping, sliced fruit, or fruit yogurt.

A tasty dessert, snack, or breakfast idea.

Nutrients per Serving

Energy	1147 kJ	Vitamin C	1 mg
	273 kcal	Calcium	142 mg
Protein	8 g	Potassium	372 mg
Fat	9 g	Iron	1.2 mg
Vitamin A	1126 IU	Zinc	0.9 mg
Folacin	25 μg	Fiber	1.9 g
Vitamin B$_{12}$	0.5 μg		

Dietary Modifications

Restricted lactose
If highly lactose intolerant, choose a bread that does not contain milk or milk solids.
Use milk treated with a commercial lactase enzyme product.
Use milk-free margarine if you are highly lactose intolerate.

Restricted fat
Omit margarine.
Replace whole milk with skim milk.

High protein
Add 80 mL ($\frac{1}{3}$ cup) skim milk powder to milk.

Restrictions

This recipe is not suitable for a restricted-fiber diet.

HIGH-ENERGY CUSTARD

6 servings

Ingredients

250 mL	Whole milk	1 cup
125 mL	Skim milk powder	$\frac{1}{2}$ cup
3	Eggs	
80 mL	Sugar	$\frac{1}{3}$ cup
0.5 mL	Salt	$\frac{1}{8}$ tsp
250 mL	Half and half cream	1 cup
3 mL	Vanilla	$\frac{3}{4}$ tsp

Preheat oven to 150°C (300°F). In a saucepan, heat milk until hot and stir in skim milk powder. In a bowl, lightly beat eggs and stir in sugar, salt, cream, and vanilla. Slowly add heated milk to egg mixture, stirring constantly. Strain into custard cups. Set into large baking pan in oven, and add boiling water to the level of custard. Bake for 45 minutes, or until knife inserted in center of custard cup comes out clean. Chill immediately.

Serving Suggestions

Serve chilled.

An excellent nutritious addition to a full fluid diet.

May be served plain or topped with a light drizzle of maple syrup or honey.

A high-energy, high-protein snack or dessert.

Nutrients per Serving

Energy	840 kJ	Vitamin C	1 mg
	200 kcal	Calcium	200 mg
Protein	9.3 g	Potassium	327 mg
Fat	9.1 g	Iron	0.5 mg
Vitamin A	170 IU	Zinc	0.9 mg
Folacin	18 μg	Fiber	0 g
Vitamin B$_{12}$	0.9 μg		

Restrictions

This recipe is unsuitable for a restricted-lactose diet or restricted-fat diet.

LEMON LOAF

1 loaf of 12 slices; 1 slice per serving

Ingredients

125 mL	Butter or margarine	$\frac{1}{2}$ cup
325 mL	Sugar	$1\frac{1}{3}$ cup
2	Eggs	
375 mL	All-purpose flour	$1\frac{1}{2}$ cups
7 mL	Baking powder	$1\frac{1}{2}$ tsp
1 mL	Salt	$\frac{1}{4}$ tsp
125 mL	Whole milk	$\frac{1}{2}$ cup
1	Lemon, rind and juice	

Preheat oven to 180°C (350°F). Grease a 21 by 11 cm (8 by 4 in) loaf pan. In a bowl, cream butter and 250 mL (1 cup) sugar. Add eggs and beat well. In a separate bowl, combine dry ingredients, mixing well. Add dry ingredients to butter mixture, alternating with milk and beating well after each addition. Stir in lemon rind. Pour batter into pan and bake for 50 to 60 minutes, or until knife inserted in center comes out clean. Blend 80 mL ($\frac{1}{3}$ cup) sugar and lemon juice while loaf is baking. Puncture baked loaf deeply with a knitting needle or similar item. Pour sugar and juice mixture over loaf while hot.

Serving Suggestions

Slice when cooled.

Serve with butter, cream cheese, or jelly.

Lemon loaf serves as a light dessert at lunch or supper.

A nice addition to a fruit and cheese tray.

Nutrients per Serving

Energy	903 kJ	Vitamin C	2 mg
	215 kcal	Calcium	46 mg
Protein	3 g	Potassium	50 mg
Fat	9.5 g	Iron	0.7 mg
Vitamin A	363 IU	Zinc	0.3 mg
Folacin	7.7 μg	Fiber	0.4 g
Vitamin B$_{12}$	0.2 μg		

Dietary Modifications

Restricted lactose
   Use milk treated with a commercial lactase enzyme product.
   Use milk-free margarine if you are highly lactose intolerate.

Restricted fat
   Choose skim milk in place of whole milk.
   Reduce butter to 80 mL ($\frac{1}{3}$ cup).

Restricted fiber
   Omit lemon rind.

High protein
   Add 50 mL ($\frac{1}{4}$ cup) skim milk powder to dry ingredients.

ZUCCHINI LOAF

2 loaves; 12 slices per loaf; 1 slice per serving

Ingredients

250 mL	Vegetable oil	1 cup
500 mL	Sugar	2 cups
3	Eggs	
625 mL	All-purpose flour	$2\frac{1}{2}$ cups
125 mL	Whole-wheat flour	$\frac{1}{2}$ cup
5 mL	Salt	1 tsp
5 mL	Baking soda	1 tsp
2.5 mL	Baking powder	$\frac{1}{2}$ tsp
500 mL	Zucchini, unpeeled, shredded	2 cups

In a bowl, beat together oil, sugar, and eggs until fluffy. In a separate bowl, combine flour, salt, and baking soda. Add wet ingredients to dry, stirring just until moistened. Gently fold in zucchini. Pour batter into two greased 23 by 13 by 7 cm (9 by 5 by 3 in) loaf pans. Bake in 180°C (350°F) oven for 1 hour and 25 minutes, or until knife inserted in center comes out clean. Cool and remove from pan.

Serving Suggestions

Bread should be allowed to cool before slicing.

Serve with soup and salad as a light lunch.

Serve buttered with a glass of chocolate milk as a snack.

Bread can be used as a light dessert to complete any meal.

An easy and different way to improve vegetable intake.

A great recipe for individuals with lactose intolerance.

Nutrients per Serving

Energy	932 kJ	Vitamin C	1 mg
	222 kcal	Calcium	19 mg
Protein	2.5 g	Potassium	69 mg
Fat	10 g	Iron	0.9 mg
Vitamin A	78 IU	Zinc	0.2 mg
Folacin	9 μg	Fiber	0.7 g
Vitamin B$_{12}$	0.1 μg		

Dietary Modifications

Restricted fiber
Replace whole-wheat flour with white flour.
Peel zucchini.

High protein
Add 50 mL ($\frac{1}{4}$ cup) skim milk powder to dry ingredients.
Increase eggs to four.

High energy
Follow high protein suggestions.

Restrictions

This recipe is unsuitable for a restricted-fat diet.

FRUIT AND FIBER LOAF

12 slices; 1 slice per serving

Ingredients

250 mL	All-purpose flour	1 cup
250 mL	Whole-wheat flour	1 cup
125 mL	Bran	½ cup
250 mL	Sugar	1 cup
250 mL	Mixed fruit, dried, chopped	1 cup
15 mL	Orange rind, grated	1 tbsp
15 mL	Baking powder	1 tbsp
5 mL	Salt	1 tsp
2	Eggs, beaten	
250 mL	Whole milk	1 cup
80 mL	Oil	⅓ cup

Preheat oven to 180°C (350°F). In a bowl, combine all dry ingredients. In a second bowl, combine all wet ingredients. Add wet ingredients to dry, stirring just until moistened. Pour mixture into greased 23 by 13 cm (9 by 5 in) loaf pan and let stand for 10 minutes. Bake 50 to 60 minutes, or until knife inserted in center comes out clean.

Serving Suggestions

Serve hot or cold.

This loaf makes an excellent breakfast snack, or accompaniment to a light lunch of cottage cheese.

An excellent fiber-containing food to aid regularity.

Nutrients per Serving

Energy	1092 kJ	Vitamin C	1 mg
	260 kcal	Calcium	94 mg
Protein	4.8 g	Potassium	218 mg
Fat	8.1 g	Iron	1.5 mg
Vitamin A	65 IU	Zinc	0.8 mg
Folacin	15 μg	Fiber	3.6 g
Vitamin B$_{12}$	0.2 μg		

Dietary Modifications

Restricted lactose
   Use milk treated with a commercial lactase enzyme product.

Restricted fat
   Use skim milk.
   Reduce oil to 50 mL ($\frac{1}{4}$ cup).

High protein
   Increase eggs to three.
   Add 50 mL ($\frac{1}{4}$ cup) skim milk powder to dry ingredients.

High energy
   Follow high protein suggestions.
   Increase oil to 125 mL ($\frac{1}{2}$ cup).

Restrictions

This recipe is not suitable for a restricted-fiber diet.

CARROT CUPCAKES

16 cupcakes; 1 cupcake per serving

Ingredients

375 mL	All-purpose flour	1½ cups
5 mL	Baking soda	1 tsp
5 mL	Baking powder	1 tsp
2 mL	Salt	½ tsp
5 mL	Cinnamon	1 tsp
250 mL	Sugar	1 cup
180 mL	Vegetable oil	¾ cup
2	Eggs	
250 mL	Carrot, raw, grated	1 cup
125 mL	Raisins	½ cup

Preheat oven to 180°C (350°F). Line muffin tins with paper baking cups. In a bowl, combine dry ingredients. In a separate bowl, beat together sugar and oil. Add eggs, one at a time, to sugar and oil mixture, beating well. Add carrots to liquid mixture. Slowly add dry ingredients to wet ingredients, stirring until blended. Stir in raisins. Divide batter into paper cups. Bake for 15 to 20 minutes, or until knife inserted in center of cupcake comes out clean.

Serving Suggestions

Allow to cool before serving.

May be iced and topped with chopped nuts.

Makes a light dessert served alone or with ice cream.

An excellent recipe if one is lactose intolerant.

Nutrients per Serving

Energy	882 kJ	Vitamin C	1 mg
	210 kcal	Calcium	34 mg
Protein	2.1 g	Potassium	80 mg

Fat	11 g	Iron	0.6 mg
Vitamin A	2070 IU	Zinc	0.2 mg
Folacin	0.6 μg	Fiber	0.8 g
Vitamin B$_{12}$	0.1 μg		

Dietary Modifications

Restricted fiber
  Omit raisins.

Restrictions

This recipe is not suitable for a restricted-fat diet.

ORANGE-CRANBERRY MUFFINS

12 medium muffins; 1 muffin per serving

Ingredients

500 mL	All-purpose flour	2 cups
160 mL	Brown sugar	$\frac{2}{3}$ cup
15 mL	Baking powder	1 tbsp
2 mL	Baking soda	$\frac{1}{2}$ tsp
2 mL	Salt	$\frac{1}{2}$ tsp
300 mL	Cranberries, frozen, chopped	$1\frac{1}{4}$ cups
2 medium	Eggs	
50 mL	Vegetable oil	$\frac{1}{4}$ cup
250 mL	2% milk	1 cup
10 mL	Orange rind, grated	2 tsp

Preheat oven to 200°C (400°F). Lightly grease 12 muffin cups. In small bowl, combine all dry ingredients. In larger bowl combine all wet ingredients. Add dry ingredients to wet, mixing just until flour is combined. Spoon batter into muffin tin, filling cups about two-thirds full. Bake for 25 minutes, or until knife inserted in center of muffin comes out clean. Remove muffins from tin and allow to cool.

Serving Suggestions

Can be served hot or cold.

Excellent served with cream cheese, jam, jelly, or preserves.

Nutrients per Serving

Energy	756 kJ	Vitamin C	2 mg
	180 kcal	Calcium	95 mg
Protein	3.9 g	Potassium	103 mg
Fat	5.2 g	Iron	1.4 mg
Vitamin A	95 IU	Zinc	0.3 mg
Folacin	10 μg	Fiber	0.7 g
Vitamin B$_{12}$	0.2 μg		

Dietary Modifications

Restricted lactose
   Use milk treated with a commercial lactase enzyme product.

High protein
   Add 50 mL ($\frac{1}{4}$ cup) skim milk powder to dry ingredients.

High energy
   Follow high protein suggestion.
   Use whole milk in place of 2% milk.
   Increase oil to 80 mL ($\frac{1}{3}$ cup).

Restrictions

This recipe is not suitable for a restricted-fiber diet.

BRAN MUFFINS

22-5 cm (2 in) muffins; 1 muffin per serving

Ingredients

500 mL	Whole-wheat flour	2 cups
375 mL	Bran	$1\frac{1}{2}$ cups
50 mL	Brown sugar	$\frac{1}{4}$ cup
1 mL	Salt	$\frac{1}{4}$ tsp
7 mL	Baking soda	$1\frac{1}{2}$ tsp
500 mL	Buttermilk	2 cups
125 mL	Molasses	$\frac{1}{2}$ cup
50 mL	Margarine, melted	$\frac{1}{4}$ cup
1	Egg, beaten	
125 mL	Raisins or dates	$\frac{1}{2}$ cup

Preheat oven to 180°C (350°F). Grease 22 muffin cups. In a bowl, combine dry ingredients, mixing well. In separate bowl, beat together wet ingredients. Add wet ingredients to dry. Lightly fold in raisins or dates. Fill muffin tins two-thirds full and bake muffins for approximately 25 minutes, or until knife inserted in center of muffin comes out clean.

Serving Suggestions

A nutritious, iron-rich breakfast alternative.

Serve with cheese and a salad to make a light lunch.

An excellent snack served with margarine, butter, jelly, cream cheese, or peanut butter.

A good source of fiber.

Nutrients per Serving

Energy	504 kJ	Vitamin C	0 μg
	120 kcal	Calcium	104 mg
Protein	3.1 g	Potassium	362 mg
Fat	2.5 g	Iron	2.5 mg
Vitamin A	92 IU	Zinc	0.6 mg
Folacin	8 μg	Fiber	2.4 g
Vitamin B$_{12}$	0.1 μg		

Dietary Modifications

Restricted lactose
   Use milk treated with a commercial lactase enzyme product.
   Use milk-free margarine if you are highly lactose intolerant.

High protein
   Increase eggs to two.
   Add 125 mL ($\frac{1}{2}$ cup) skim milk powder to dry ingredients.

High energy
   Follow high protein suggestions.
   Increase margarine to 80 mL ($\frac{1}{3}$ cup).

Restrictions

This recipe is not suitable for a restricted-fiber diet.

BANANA-CAROB PEANUT BUTTER MUFFINS

10 medium muffins; 1 muffin per serving

Ingredients

250 mL	All-purpose flour	1 cup
125 mL	Whole wheat flour	$\frac{1}{2}$ cup
15 mL	Baking powder	1 tbsp
2 mL	Baking soda	$\frac{1}{2}$ tsp
2 mL	Salt	$\frac{1}{2}$ tsp
2 medium	Eggs, slightly beaten	
125 mL	Honey	$\frac{1}{2}$ cup
125 mL	Vegetable oil	$\frac{1}{2}$ cup
2 medium	Bananas, mashed	
125 mL	Peanut butter, crunchy	$\frac{1}{2}$ cup
80 mL	Carob chips	$\frac{1}{3}$ cup

Preheat oven to 200°C (400°F). Grease 10 muffin cups. In small bowl, combine all dry ingredients. In larger bowl, combine all wet ingredients. Add dry ingredients to wet, folding gently until flour is just moistened. Spoon batter into muffin tin, filling cups about two-thirds full. Bake for 20 minutes, or until knife inserted in center of muffin comes out clean. Remove muffins from tin and allow to cool.

Serving Suggestions

Can be served hot or cold.

Serve plain or spread with butter, peanut butter, or jam.

An excellent snack idea.

The peanut butter adds extra protein.

A good recipe if one is lactose intolerant.

Nutrients per Serving

Energy	1554 kJ	Vitamin C	2 mg
	370 kcal	Calcium	31 mg
Protein	7.7 g	Potassium	268 mg
Fat	21 g	Iron	1.4 mg
Vitamin A	79 IU	Zinc	0.8 mg
Folacin	26 μg	Fiber	2.4 g
Vitamin B$_{12}$	0.1 μg		

Restrictions

This recipe is not suitable for a restricted-fat diet or restricted-fiber diet.

PEACHY STRAWBERRY CHEESECAKE PIE

8 servings

Ingredients

375 g	Cream cheese, softened	9 oz
2	Eggs	
180 mL	Sugar	$\frac{3}{4}$ cup
5 mL	Vanilla	1 tsp
1	Graham cracker pie shell, unbaked	
125 mL	Sour cream	$\frac{1}{2}$ cup
250 mL	Strawberries, fresh, halved	1 cup
250 mL	Peaches, fresh, sliced	1 cup
125 mL	Strawberry or peach jelly	$\frac{1}{2}$ cup
80 mL	Coconut, grated, toasted	$\frac{1}{3}$ cup

Preheat oven to 180°C (350°F). In a bowl, beat cream cheese until smooth. Add eggs, sugar, and vanilla, beating well to combine. Pour mixture into pie shell. Bake for 35 to 40 minutes, or until knife inserted in center comes out clean. Remove from oven and spread with sour cream. Allow pie to cool completely. Arrange fruit on top of pie. In a small saucepan, melt jelly. Spoon jelly over fruit. Sprinkle with coconut. Chill pie well before serving.

Serving Suggestions

Serve chilled alone or accompanied by ice cream.

A very attractive dessert to serve to guests.

Various combinations of other fruits can be used.

Nutrients per Serving

Energy	2037 kJ	Vitamin C	14 mg
	485 kcal	Calcium	77 mg
Protein	7.3 g	Potassium	272 mg
Fat	27 g	Iron	1.4 mg

Vitamin A	1094 IU	Zinc	0.8 mg
Folacin	17 μg	Fiber	3.1 g
Vitamin B$_{12}$	0.4 μg		

Dietary Modifications

Restricted fiber
Omit strawberries and replace with sliced honeydew melon.
Remove skin from peaches.
Omit coconut and replace with candy sprinkles.

Restrictions

This recipe is not suitable for a restricted-lactose diet or restricted-fat diet.

PEANUT BUTTER SURPRISE PIE

8 servings

Ingredients

80 mL	Peanut butter, crunchy	$\frac{1}{3}$ cup
80 mL	Corn syrup	$\frac{1}{3}$ cup
50 mL	Chocolate chips	$\frac{1}{4}$ cup
500 mL	Crisp rice cereal	2 cups
1 medium	Banana, thinly sliced	
1 L	Vanilla ice cream, softened	1 qt
50 mL	Coconut, toasted	$\frac{1}{4}$ cup

Lightly grease a 23 cm (9 in) pie pan. In bowl, mix together peanut butter and syrup. Stir in chocolate chips and cereal. To form crust of pie, firmly pack peanut butter mixture into pie pan, spreading evenly. Chill crust in freezer until firm. Remove crust and line with banana slices. Evenly spread softened ice cream over banana layer. Sprinkle with toasted coconut. Return to freezer until firm.

Serving Suggestions

Allow pie to thaw for a few minutes before cutting.

This recipe is an excellent dessert for company.

The peanut butter provides a high-protein content.

Nutrients per Serving

Energy	1554 kJ	Vitamin C	6 mg
	370 kcal	Calcium	99 mg
Protein	6 g	Potassium	280 mg
Fat	20 g	Iron	1.4 mg
Vitamin A	819 IU	Zinc	1.2 mg
Folacin	31 μg	Fiber	0.6 g
Vitamin B$_{12}$	0.3 μg		

Restrictions

This recipe is not suitable for a restricted-lactose diet, restricted-fat diet, or restricted-fiber diet.

RHUBARB CAKE

8 servings

Ingredients

125 mL	Margarine	$\frac{1}{2}$ cup
375 mL	Brown sugar	$1\frac{1}{2}$ cups
1 medium	Egg	
250 mL	Buttermilk	1 cup
5 mL	Vanilla	1 tsp
500 mL	All-purpose flour	2 cups
5 mL	Baking soda	1 tsp
pinch	Salt	
375 mL	Rhubarb, raw, finely chopped	$1\frac{1}{2}$ cups
50 mL	Sugar	$\frac{1}{4}$ cup
5 mL	Cinnamon	1 tsp
125 mL	Walnuts, chopped	$\frac{1}{2}$ cup

Heat oven to 180°C (350°F). In a bowl, cream together margarine and brown sugar. Blend in egg, buttermilk, and vanilla. In separate bowl, combine flour, baking soda, and salt. Add flour mixture to sugar and milk mixture, blending well. Stir in rhubarb. Pour batter into a well-greased 23 cm (9 in) square pan. Combine cinnamon and sugar and sprinkle on top of batter. Top with chopped nuts. Bake for 45 to 50 minutes, or until knife inserted in center comes out clean.

Serving Suggestions

Serve hot or cold.

Excellent topped with whipped cream or accompanied by ice cream.

A delicious dessert or snack idea.

Nuts can be omitted if desired.

Nutrients per Serving

Energy	1827 kJ	Vitamin C	2 mg
	435 kcal	Calcium	122 mg
Protein	7.4 g	Potassium	309 mg

Fat	18 g	Iron	2.9 mg
Vitamin A	586 IU	Zinc	0.8 mg
Folacin	19 μg	Fiber	1.6 g
Vitamin B$_{12}$	0.1 μg		

Dietary Modifications

Restricted lactose
   Use milk treated with a commercial lactase enzyme product.
   Use milk-free margarine if you are highly lactose intolerant.

High protein
   Add 50 mL ($\frac{1}{4}$ cup) skim milk powder to dry ingredients.
   Increase eggs to two.

Restrictions

This recipe is unsuitable for a restricted-fat diet or restricted-fiber diet.

ROLLED OAT CAKE WITH MOCHA ICING

8 servings

Ingredients—Cake

250 mL	Rolled oats	1 cup
375 mL	Water, boiling	1½ cups
125 mL	Butter	½ cup
250 mL	Brown sugar, packed	1 cup
5 mL	Vanilla	1 tsp
250 mL	All-purpose flour	1 cup
5 mL	Baking soda	1 tsp
2 mL	Salt	½ tsp
250 mL	Dates, chopped	1 cup
125 mL	Walnuts, chopped	½ cup

Ingredients—Icing

30 mL	Butter	2 tbsp
300 mL	Icing sugar	1¼ cups
30 mL	Cocoa	2 tbsp
pinch	Salt	
15 mL	Coffee, black	1 tbsp
5 mL	Vanilla	1 tsp

Preheat oven to 180°C (350°F). Lightly grease a 23 cm (9 in) square pan. In a small bowl, combine oats and boiling water and cool. In a larger bowl, cream together butter and sugar until fluffy. Add cooled mixture and vanilla to butter mixture, beating well. In a bowl, stir together flour, baking soda, and salt. Stir in dates and nuts. Add dry ingredients to wet, beating well to blend. Pour batter into pan and bake for 35 minutes or until done. Cool cake in pan. Make icing by creaming together margarine and sugar. Stir in remaining ingredients, adding more coffee if icing is too stiff to spread easily. Ice cooled cake.

Serving Suggestions

Serve plain or iced, alone or with ice cream.

An excellent dessert or snack.

Nutrients per Serving

Energy	2251 kJ	Vitamin C	0 mg
	536 kcal	Calcium	77 mg
Protein	6.2 g	Potassium	362 mg
Fat	20 g	Iron	2.8 mg
Vitamin A	650 IU	Zinc	0.8 mg
Folacin	17 μg	Fiber	4.1 g
Vitamin B_{12}	0 μg		

Dietary Modifications

Restricted Lactose
Use milk-free margarine if you are highly lactose intolerant.

Restrictions

This recipe is not suitable for a restricted-fat or restricted-fiber diet.

APPLE-RHUBARB CRISP

6 servings

Ingredients

500 mL	Apples, tart, sliced, peeled	2 cups
500 mL	Rhubarb, fresh, cubed	2 cups
300 mL	Sugar	$1\frac{1}{3}$ cups
125 mL	All-purpose flour	$\frac{1}{2}$ cup
125 mL	Rolled oats	$\frac{1}{2}$ cup
2 mL	Cinnamon	$\frac{1}{2}$ tsp
50 mL	Butter or margarine	$\frac{1}{4}$ cup

Heat oven to 190°C (375°F). Grease a 20 cm (8 in) square baking pan. Place apples and rhubarb in pan. Combine remaining ingredients and sprinkle over fruit. Bake for 30 to 40 minutes or until golden brown.

Serving Suggestions

Serve warm or cold with ice cream.

A quick, easy nutritious dessert.

An excellent recipe if one is lactose intolerant.

Nutrients per Serving

Energy	1315 kJ	Vitamin C	6 mg
	315 kcal	Calcium	47 mg
Protein	2.7 g	Potassium	206 mg
Fat	7.3 g	Iron	0.8 mg
Vitamin A	315 IU	Zinc	0.4 mg
Folacin	8 μg	Fiber	2.5 g
Vitamin B_{12}	0 μg		

Dietary Modifications

Restricted Lactose
    Use milk-free margarine if you are highly lactose intolerant.

Restricted fat
    Reduce butter to 30 mL (2 tbsp).

High energy
    Increase butter to 80 mL ($\frac{1}{3}$ cup).

Restrictions

This recipe is unsuitable for a restricted-fiber diet.

GRANOLA BARS

8 bars; 1 bar per serving

Ingredients

500 mL	Granola	2 cups
2 medium	Eggs, beaten	

In a bowl, mix together granola and eggs. Spread mixture in greased 20 cm (8 in) square pan. Bake in 180°C (350°F) oven for 15 minutes. When cooled, cut into eight bars.

Serving Suggestions

A nutritious, high-energy snack idea.

Nutrients per Serving

Energy	735 kJ	Vitamin C	0 mg
	175 kcal	Calcium	25 mg
Protein	5.3 g	Potassium	175 mg
Fat	9.8 g	Iron	1.4 mg
Vitamin A	80 IU	Zinc	1.3 mg
Folacin	3 μg	Fiber	1.4 g
Vitamin B$_{12}$	0.1 μg		

Restrictions

This recipe is unsuitable for a restricted-fat or restricted-fiber diet.

ANITA'S PEANUT BUTTER COOKIES

36 cookies; 2 cookies per serving

Ingredients

125 mL	Whole-wheat flour	$\frac{1}{2}$ cup
125 mL	All-purpose flour	$\frac{1}{2}$ cup
50 mL	Soybean flour	$\frac{1}{4}$ cup
2 mL	Salt	$\frac{1}{2}$ tsp
2 mL	Baking soda	$\frac{1}{2}$ tsp
125 mL	Sugar	$\frac{1}{2}$ cup
125 mL	Butter or margarine	$\frac{1}{2}$ cup
125 mL	Brown sugar	$\frac{1}{2}$ cup
1	Egg	
125 mL	Peanut butter, crunchy	$\frac{1}{2}$ cup
2 mL	Vanilla	$\frac{1}{2}$ tsp

Preheat oven to 180°C (350°F). Combine all dry ingredients except sugar, and set aside. In a bowl, cream butter. Beat sugar into butter, adding a little at a time. Add egg, one at a time, beating well. Add peanut butter and vanilla, mixing well. Slowly add dry ingredients to wet. Shape into 2.5 cm (1 in) balls and place on ungreased cookie sheet. (Leave space for spreading.) Press flat with a floured fork or the bottom of a floured glass. Bake for 10 minutes or until lightly browned.

Serving Suggestions

Serve alone or with ice cream as a dessert or snack.

A handful of nuts, seeds or carob chips can be added for additional flavor and texture.

Nutrients per Serving

Energy	693 kJ	Vitamin C	0 mg
	165 kcal	Calcium	16 mg
Protein	3.8 g	Potassium	102 mg
Fat	9.6 g	Iron	0.6 mg

Vitamin A	216 IU	Zinc	0.3 mg
Folacin	13 μg	Fiber	0.4 g
Vitamin B$_{12}$	0.1 μg		

Dietary Modifications

Resticted lactose
Use milk-free margarine if you are highly lactose intolerant.

High protein
Add 50 mL ($\frac{1}{4}$ cup) skim milk powder to dry ingredients.

Restrictions

This recipe is not suitable for a restricted-fat or restricted-fiber diet.

13

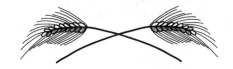

Sample Weekly Menu

SAMPLE MENU

Monday			
Breakfast	Milk	250 mL	1 cup
	Oven French Toast* topped with	2 slices	
	Sliced canned peaches	125 mL	½ cup
Lunch	Tomato juice	250 mL	1 cup
	Chicken-Rice Soup*	1 serving	
	Whole-wheat dinner roll with	1 small	
	Margarine	10 mL	2 tsp
	Fruit Yogurt*	1 serving	
Snack	Apple juice	125 mL	½ cup
Evening meal	Milk	250 mL	1 cup
	Stir Fry Beef with Vegetables*	1 serving	
	Boiled white rice	250 mL	1 cup
	Orange sherbet topped with	125 mL	½ cup
	Sliced banana	½ medium	
Snack	Toasted raisin bread with	1 slice	
	Peanut butter	15 mL	1 tbsp
Tuesday			
Breakfast	High Protein Nog*	1 serving	
	Toasted whole-wheat bread with	1 slice	
	Margarine	5 mL	1 tsp
Snack	Orange juice	125 mL	½ cup
	Crackers with	6	
	Peanut butter	30 mL	2 tbsp
Lunch	Milk	250 mL	1 cup
	Chili*	1 serving	
	Cornbread* with	1 square	
	Margarine	5 mL	1 tsp
Evening meal	Tossed side salad with	125 mL	½ cup
	French dressing	15 mL	1 tbsp
	Baked Salmon Squares*	1 serving	
	Canned peas	125 mL	½ cup
	Mashed potatoes	125 mL	½ cup
	Fresh apple	1 average	
Snack	Fruit and Fiber Loaf*	1 slice	
	Pineapple juice	125 mL	½ cup

* Recipes for these dishes found in the recipe section

(Continued)

SAMPLE MENU *(Continued)*

	Wednesday		
Breakfast	Fresh grapefruit topped with	$\frac{1}{2}$ medium	
	Brown sugar	15 mL	1 tbsp
	Tasty Breakfast Treat*	1 serving	
Lunch	Milk	250 mL	1 cup
	Cool and Creamy Carrot Soup*	1 serving	
	Ritz® crackers	6	
	Oatmeal cookies	2	
Snack	Monkey Mapleshake*	1 serving	
Evening meal	Milk	125 mL	$\frac{1}{2}$ cup
	Hamburger pattie	1 medium	
	Brussels sprouts	125 mL	$\frac{1}{2}$ cup
	Boiled potato with	1 medium	
	Margarine	5 mL	1 tsp
	Fruit gelatin	125 mL	$\frac{1}{2}$ cup
Snack	Pita bread stuffed with	$\frac{1}{2}$ pita	
	Chopped ham salad and	125 mL	$\frac{1}{2}$ cup
	Shredded lettuce	125 mL	$\frac{1}{2}$ cup
	Thursday		
Brunch	Orange juice	125 mL	$\frac{1}{2}$ cup
	Creamy High-Protein Omelet*	1 serving	
	Toasted white bread with	2 slices	
	Margarine	15 mL	1 tbsp
	Fresh fruit	125 mL	$\frac{1}{2}$ cup
Snack	Crackers with	6	
	Cream cheese	30 mL	2 tbsp
Evening meal	Vegetable juice	125 mL	$\frac{1}{2}$ cup
	Citrus Chicken*	1 serving	
	Steamed white rice	125 mL	$\frac{1}{2}$ cup
	Steamed carrots with	125 mL	$\frac{1}{2}$ cup
	Margarine	5 mL	1 tsp
	Apple	1 medium	
Snack	Milk	250 mL	1 cup
	Digestive cookies	2	

(Continued)

SAMPLE MENU *(Continued)*

	Friday		
Breakfast	Orange juice	125 mL	$\frac{1}{2}$ cup
	Toasted white bread with	2 slices	
	Peanut butter	30 mL	2 tbsp
Snack	Fresh pear	1 medium	
Lunch	Milk	250 mL	1 cup
	Sunshine Salad*	1 serving	
	Whole-wheat dinner roll with	1 medium	
	Margarine	5 mL	1 tsp
Snack	Butterscotch pudding	125 mL	$\frac{1}{2}$ cup
Evening meal	Tomato juice	125 mL	$\frac{1}{2}$ cup
	Milk	250 mL	1 cup
	Clam Casserole*	1 serving	
	Steamed broccoli	125 mL	$\frac{1}{2}$ cup
	Fruit gelatin	125 mL	$\frac{1}{2}$ cup
Snack	Cheddar cheese and	45 g	$1\frac{1}{2}$ oz
	Crackers	6	

	Saturday		
Breakfast	Grapefruit juice	125 mL	$\frac{1}{2}$ cup
	Cottage cheese topped with	125 mL	$\frac{1}{2}$ cup
	Fresh sliced strawberries	50 mL	$\frac{1}{4}$ cup
	Toasted English muffin with	1	
	Jelly	10 mL	2 tsp
Lunch	Milk	250 mL	1 cup
	Filling Fish Soup*	1 serving	
	Buttered French bread	1 thick slice	
	Apple	1 medium	
Snack	Whole-wheat bread with	1 slice	
	Honey	15 mL	1 tbsp
Evening meal	Tossed green salad with	250 mL	1 cup
	Oil and vinegar dressing	30 mL	2 tbsp
	Baked pork chop	1 small	
	Orange-Raisin Rice*	1 serving	
	Canned green beans with	125 mL	$\frac{1}{2}$ cup
	Margarine	5 mL	1 tsp
Snack	Plain yogurt sweetened with	180 mL	$\frac{3}{4}$ cup
	Maple syrup	15 mL	1 tbsp

(Continued)

SAMPLE MENU *(Continued)*

	Sunday		
Brunch	Orange-pineapple juice	125 mL	$\frac{1}{2}$ cup
	Crustless Quiche*	1 serving	
	Whole-wheat scones with	1 scone	
	Margarine	10 mL	2 tsp
	Fresh fruit cup	125 mL	$\frac{1}{2}$ cup
Snack	Milk	250 mL	1 cup
	Plain muffin with	1 medium	
	Margarine	5 mL	1 tsp
Evening meal	Vegetable juice	125 mL	$\frac{1}{2}$ cup
	Waldorf Salad*	1 serving	
	Roast beef	90 g	3 oz
	Baked potato with	1 medium	
	Sour cream	30 mL	2 tbsp
	Baked squash, mashed with	125 mL	$\frac{1}{2}$ cup
	Butter	5 mL	1 tsp
Snack	Milk	250 mL	1 cup
	Anita's Peanut Butter Cookies*	2	

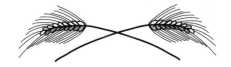

Resource Guide

In order to understand the importance of good nutrition, a sound knowledge of the many aspects of IBD is required. The following is a list of available resources that provide such information.

NATIONAL IBD SUPPORT ORGANIZATIONS

The following are nonprofit organizations dedicated to finding the cause and a cure for IBD by funding medical research and educational programs. They strive to improve the treatment of individuals with IBD and to provide current information on the disease for individuals and their families, health professionals, and the general public. Contact the national office to locate the nearest chapter in your area.

The Canadian Foundation for Ileitis and Colitis, National Office
21 St. Clair Avenue East, Suite 301
Toronto, Ontario, Canada. M4T 1L9
(416) 920-5035
The Crohn's and Colitis Foundation of America, National Office
444 Park Avenue South, 11th floor
New York, NY, 10016–7374
(212) 685-3440
(Formerly the National Foundation for Ileitis and Colitis.)

Other Organizations

The Oley Foundation
214 Hun Memorial, Albany Medical Center
Albany, NY, 12208 (518) 445-5079

This nonprofit organization was established in 1983 to address the special needs of individuals on home nutrition support, both enteral and parenteral. One of the foundation's commitments is to enhance the quality of life and functional status of these individuals. The objectives of this foundation encompass research, training, and education. For consumers, a bimonthly publication, entitled the "Lifeline Letter," is available and includes articles written by health care workers or individuals on home nutrition support. Although not specifically directed at individuals with IBD, the information is pertinent to any individual who must receive home nutrition support.

BOOKS

Idiopathic Inflammatory Bowel Disease: Crohn's Disease and Chronic Ulcerative Colitis. Edited by Dr. A. B. R. Thomson for the Canadian Foundation for Ileitis and Colitis. Published by the Canadian Public Health Association, 1982. Written for health care professionals and individuals with IBD and their families, the book provides a comprehensive review of the subject of IBD. Topics covered include clinical features, etiology and pathogenesis, diagnosis, complications, and management. Available from the Canadian Foundation for Ileitis and Colitis at a price of $15.00 (price may vary).

People... Not Patients: A Source Book for Living with Inflammatory Bowel Disease. Edited by P. Steiner, P. Banks, D. Present. Published through the Crohn's and Colitis Foundation of America, 1985. Written for individuals with IBD, it provides information on medical aspects such as diagnosis and medications, practical advice on diet and exercise, and available educational material. Available from the Crohn's and Colitis Foundation of America and also from the Canadian Foundation for Ileitis and Colitis. Price: $40.00 (price may vary).

The Crohn's Disease and Ulcerative Colitis Fact Book. Edited by P. Banks, D. Present, P. Steiner. Published through the Crohn's and Colitis Foundation of America, 1983. Written for individuals with IBD. Part I reviews epidemiology and diagnosis. Other sections include medical, nutritional, and surgical treatment as well as practical information on living with the disease. Available from the Crohn's and Colitis Foundation of America as well as the Canadian Foundation for Ileitis and Colitis. Price: $20.00 (price may vary).

A Special Kind of Cookbook, 2nd Ed. Edited by Mary Sue Waisman. Published by The Canadian Foundation for Ileitis and Colitis, 1989. Written for individuals with IBD, this book is mainly a cookbook, but contains short informative discussions of normal nutrition, dietary modifications, and other relevant information. Available from the Canadian Foundation for Ileitis and Colitis. Price: $10.00 (price may vary).

REGISTERED DIETITIAN

Many individuals claim to be nutrition professionals, but they may lack the credentials and thus be unqualified to provide nutrition information. You are encouraged to seek out a competent and qualified registered dietitian (R.D.) to provide you with current nutrition information and to counsel you regarding dietary modifications. A registered dietitian (R.D.) is an individual who has obtained a university degree in foods and nutrition (or a related field) and who has successfully completed an internship program at an accredited institution. In some provinces and states, receipients of a master's degree or Ph.D. in nutrition may be granted the use of the credentials of a registered dietitian. Only those individuals who have fulfilled these requirements may use the professional title of registered dietitian and use the initials R.D. (Some provinces also use the initials R.P.Dt., R.D.N., or P.Dt.). If you are a patient in a hospital or attending an outpatient clinic affiliated with a hospital, the nutrition expert will be a registered dietitian. If you are in the community and want to locate a registered dietitian in private practice, the initials R.D. (or as noted above) will ensure that the individual is qualified. You are encouraged to contact the local dietetic association for a list of registered dietitians in private practice. The association will be listed in the telephone directory.

SERVICES AVAILABLE TO PROVIDE
NUTRITION ADVICE

Hospital-based outpatient registered dietitian. This service is offered by many hospitals in both the United States and Canada to provide individualized nutrition counseling for individuals in the community. Contact your local hospital regarding available services.

Hospital inpatient registered dietitian. If you are a patient in a Canadian or U.S. hospital, a registered dietitian will often be involved in your care. He or she will answer nutrition questions and provide individualized nutrition counseling. If you are in the hospital but are not working with a dietitian, ask the health care staff for a referral.

Community nutritionist. Although a limited service, local health units or departments may be contacted to provide nutrition information. The ability to provide individualized counseling varies with the unit. To locate the nearest health unit, refer to your local telephone directory.

Private practice registered dietitian. Some states and provinces have nutrition professionals that provide individualized nutrition counseling on a fee-for-service basis. To locate a private practice registered dietitian, contact the local professional dietetic association for a listing.

Dial-a-dietitian. In Canada, this free public service is offered by several provincial professional dietetic associations. Nutrition-related questions can be phoned in and will be answered by a registered dietitian. Generally, no individualized nutrition counseling is provided. Consult the telephone directory for the phone number.

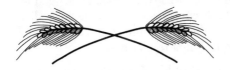

Glossary

Acute   Sudden onset of disease associated with severe symptoms.

Amino Acid   The basic unit that makes up protein.

Anemia   A reduction in hemoglobin or insufficient red blood cells.

Anorexia   A lack of appetite for food.

Antibodies   Blood components that fight infection.

Antibiotics   A substance that destroys or interferes with the growth of microorganisms.

Antioxidant   Agents that bind with oxygen to prevent unwanted changes.

Aerophagia   The habit of swallowing air.

Basic Four   In the United States, the food guide used to help individuals balance their diet. Foods are divided into four food groups; the number of servings and the serving sizes that should be consumed on a regular basis are outlined.

Calorie   *See* kilocalorie.

Canada's Food Guide   In Canada, the food guide used to help individuals balance their diet to meet nutrient needs. The guide divides food into four food groups and outlines the number of servings and the serving sizes that should be consumed on a regular basis.

Capillary   A tiny, thin-walled blood vessel that connects the smallest arteries with the smallest veins.

Catabolism   The series of chemical reactions that take place in the body in which complex substances are broken down to simpler substances and energy is released.

Colectomy   The surgical removal of the colon.

Colostomy   The creation of a surgical passage through the wall of the abdomen to a section of the colon.

Collagen   A protein substance found in all fibrous tissue including connective tissue, cartilage, and skin.

Colon   The large intestine.

Constipation   The irregular, difficult, or sluggish passage of stool.

Corticosteroid   A class of medications used to reduce inflammation. Example: prednisone.

Crohn's Disease   A chronic progressive inflammatory disease of unknown etiology. The disease can affect any section of the gastrointestinal tract from mouth to anus and involve all layers of the bowel wall. Involvement of the terminal ileum is common. Complications such as fistulae may develop.

Chronic   Recurring or occurring over a long period of time.

Defecation   Evacuation of the bowels.

Diarrhea   A deviation from usual bowel habits highlighted by the presence of frequent loose stools.

Diverticular Disease   Herniations or outpouchings of the wall of the gastrointestinal tract.

Duodenum   The first portion of the small intestine.

Edema   The collection of unusually large amounts of body fluid in a part of, or all of, the body; causes swelling.

Elemental Formula   A specially designed, nutritionally complete product that contains nutrients in their simplest form. This product requires little digestion and is easily absorbed in the upper section of the small intestine. It is often referred to as predigested formula.

Energy   The fuel required by the body to power body processes. Energy is obtained from carbohydrate, protein, and fat.

Enterstomal Therapy Nurse   A nurse that specializes in the care of ostomies.

Enzyme   A protein that facilitates chemical reactions.

Excretion   Elimination from the body.

Feces   Waste matter excreted from the bowel consisting of unabsorbed food, water, bacteria, and intestinal secretions.

Fiber   That portion of a plant that the human body cannot digest. It provides undigestible bulk, which encourages the normal elimination of body wastes.

Fissure   An ulcer, crack, or furrow in a body organ.

Fistula   An abnormal tubelike communication between two body surfaces or cavities.

Gastrointestinal Tract   The organ of nutrient digestion and absorption extending from the mouth to the anus.

Gastrostomy Tube Feeding   The delivery of a liquid nutritional formula into the stomach through a feeding tube inserted into the wall of the stomach.

Goal Weight   A realistic individualized weight. Often a compromise between ideal weight and usual weight.

Good Nutrition   The state that exists when the body has been receiving the required amounts of the nutrients it needs to function properly.

Hemoglobin   The red blood cell constituent that transports oxygen and carbon dioxide.

Ideal Body Weight   The recommended weight for height and age that is associated with good health.

Ileostomy   A surgically created opening from the surface of the body to the ileum.

Inflammation   The reaction of living tissue to irritation, infection, or injury characterized by swelling, pain, heat, and redness, with the possible loss or reduction of function.

Inflammatory Bowel Disease   Refers to the two chronic inflammatory conditions of Crohn's disease and ulcerative colitis.

Ileum   The last section of the small bowel. Located between the jejunum and the colon.

Jejunum   That portion of the small bowel located between the duodenum and the ileum.

Kilocalorie   A measurement of the release of energy from food. Often the term *calorie* is incorrectly used in place of this term.

Kilojoule   A System International (SI) or metric measurement of the release of energy from food. One kilocalorie equals 4.18 kilojoules.

Lactose   The natural sugar found in milk.

Lactose Intolerance   The inability to digest and absorb lactose due to an insufficient amount of lactase in the gastrointestinal tract.

Macronutrients   Nutrients required in relatively large amounts.

Malabsorption   Poor or disordered absorption.

Malnutrition   The state of being poorly nourished.

Megaloblastic Anemia   A type of anemia that is characterized by abnormally large red blood cells.

Metabolism   The sum total of all chemical reactions that take place in living cells.

Micronutrients   Nutrients required in relatively small amounts.

Mineral   An element in a simple inorganic form.

Nasogastric Tube Feeding   The delivery of nutrition to the gastrointestinal tract through a tube inserted through the nasal passage and into the stomach.

Nutrition   The relationship of food to the well-being of the body.

Nutrients   The chemical components of food that the body requires to perform the various activities associated with living.

Osteoporosis   A condition where the density of bone decreases, causing the bone to become weaker and more susceptible to fractures.

Osteomalacia   A condition in which there is a softening of the bone, leading to deformities.

Oxidation   The process by which the tissues of the body make the energy in food available to the body.

Parenteral Nutrition   The delivery of nutrients to the body through a vein.

Peptide   A short chain of amino acids.

Protein-energy Malnutrition   A deficiency of both protein and energy leading to weight loss, poor healing, and reduced resistance to infection. Often referred to as protein-calorie malnutrition.

Protein-losing Enteropathy   Loss of protein through the inflamed bowel wall.

Recommended Nutrient Intake (RNI)   In Canada, the level of dietary intake of essential nutrients considered to be adequate to meet the nutritional needs of most healthy individuals as based on age, sex, body size, activity, and diet.

Recommended Dietary Allowance (RDA)   In the United States, the level of dietary intake of essential nutrients considered to be sufficient to meet the nutritional needs of most healthy individuals based on age, sex, body size, activity and diet.

Registered Dietitian   A nutrition professional qualified through education and mandatory recognized professional affiliation to participate, advise, and direct in the field of nutrition.

Relapse   The reinitiation of active disease after a period of inactive disease.

Remission   The period in which disease is inactive.

Resection   Surgical excision.

Steatorrhea   Excessive fat in the stool.

Stool   Fecal discharge from the bowel.

Stricture   The abnormal narrowing of a passage due to scar tissue.

Subcutaneous Fat   The layer of fat just under the skin.

Synthesis   The process that involves the formation of a complex substance from a simpler substance. For example, the building of protein from amino acids.

Terminal Ileum   The end section of the small intestine.

Tube Feeding   The delivery of nutrients to the gastrointestinal tract through a tube.

Underweight   A weight less than 90% of ideal weight for height, age, and body build.

Ulcerative Colitis   A chronic inflammatory condition of unknown etiology that affects the large intestine; always involves the rectum. Unlike Crohn's disease, it generally involves only the mucosa.

Vegan   Strict vegetarians who avoid all animal-source foods.

Vitamin   An organic substance required by the body in trace amounts for normal metabolic functioning.

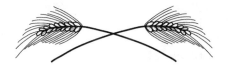

Index